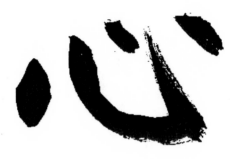

Kokoro . . . Mind / Heart

CALLIGRAPHY BY MASAHIRO OKI

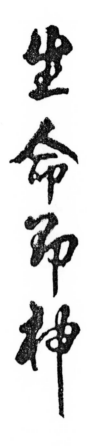

Your Lifeforce is God.

CALLIGRAPHY BY MASAHIRO OKI

Masahiro Oki

The Joy of Yoga

CREATING HEALTH & BEAUTY

IN BODY, MIND & SPIRIT

TRANSLATED AND EDITED BY

Kazuko Tatsumura Hillyer, PhD, OMD

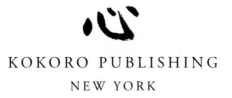

KOKORO PUBLISHING

NEW YORK

Kokoro Publishing
20 West 64th Street, #24E
New York City NY 10023
Tel. No. (212) 799-9711
Fax. No. (212) 799-1661
Email: info@gaiaholistic.com

The exercises and practices in *The Joy of Yoga* are not intended to replace
the services of your physician or to provide an alternative to professional
medical treatment. *The Joy of Yoga* offers no diagnosis of or treatment for
any specific medical problem that you may have. Where it suggests the
possible usefulness of certain practices in relation to certain physical
problems or mental condition, it does so solely for educational
purposes—either to explore the possible relationship of natural
breathing to health, or to expose the reader to alternative
health and healing approaches.

Printed in the United States

ISBN 978-0-9704979-5-6

Designed by Dede Cummings
Edited by Ellen Keelan; production by Carolyn Kasper / dcdesign
Cover art concept by Kazuko Tatsumura Hillyer, PhD, OMD

The cover design represents the planet earth ("Gaia"), with the top
representing blue sky and sunlight; the middle section,
green trees; the brown, earth itself; and the red,
the magma beneath the ground.

This printer supports the Tree Program and uses recycled paper.

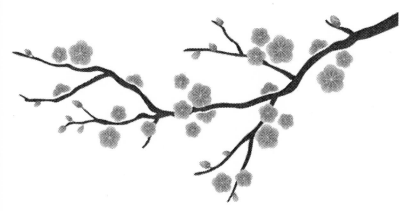

Our thanks to Masahiro Oki who taught us a path.

Acknowledgments

On behalf of Kokoro Publishing, I extend my deepest gratitude to the following people who have inspired me deeply and encouraged me to publish the series of nine books on Health and Spirituality

To my spiritual teachers: His Holiness the 14 Dalai Lama and Mother Theresa

To my masters, the late Masahiro Oki, the late Masato Nakagawa, and the late Tomeko Mitsui.

To Rev. Mikinosuke Kakizaka, the head abbot of Tenkawa Shinko Shrine.

To Osamu Tatsumura, Fernando and Paula Montoto and many other colleagues who has always helped me tirelessly.

With deepest gratitude and Compassion,
Kazuko Tatsumura PhD, OMD, October 2010

Preface

Although my encounter and studies with Master Oki were rather short and scattered into the span of about 10 years from 1970 till his passing in 1985, they were always intense and very powerful. His influence on me is still very vivid, and continuous to this day, or rather till the end of my life.

This book is the fifth in a series of nine books on health and spirituality being published by Kokoro Publishing. The series includes the following titles:

- *Overcoming Cancer and Other Difficult Diseases in a Holistic Way*, by Tomeko Mitsui and Kazuko Tatsumura Hillyer (published in 2003, second edition in 2007)

- *Your Immune Revolution* and *Healing Your Healing Power*, by Toru Abo & Kazuko Tatsumura Hillyer (published in 2007)

- *Deep Breath Changes Your Body and Mind/Spirit*, by Osamu Tatsumura (published in 2008)

- *Mystery of the Body's Relationship: Kanrenbui*, by Fernando and Paula Montoto (published in 2009)

- *Joy of Yoga*, by Masahiro Oki (published in 2010)

I hope you enjoy these books. We would love to hear your comments. Please feel free to contact me at 212-799-9711, fax 212-799-1661, or email me at kazuko@gaiaholistic.com. or visit www.gaiaholistic.com for any comments or more information, or how to purchase these books.

With deep gratitude and Compassion,
Kazuko Tatsumura Hillyer, PhD., OMD

Contents

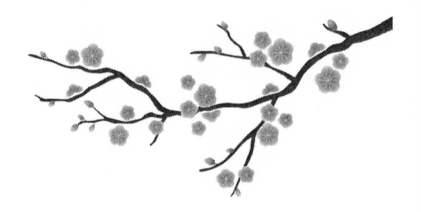

Introduction

Yoga Releases Your Mind and Body from Worry

Y O G A is the most effective method for beauty and health

Yoga can fix most of our emotional and physical problems. It can even make your wishes come true: losing weight, looking prettier, growing taller, becoming more intelligent, overcoming neuroses, and so on. This extraordinary effect has made yoga extremely popular not only in Japan but all over the world.

People suffer from many problems today. Their lungs can't breathe well after going up thirty stairs, their uterus can't deliver a child without the help of others, and when their stomach feels bad they think it's cancer. All year they complain about their body's malfunctions. I've heard that in the U.S. obesity is considered a sign of poverty, which is the direct opposite of traditional notions of obesity, and that people take vitamin pills religiously to lose weight. It's totally unhealthy.

It's natural that our minds and bodies are out of balance, because our "civilized" lifestyle is contrary to the natural way of living. And, as social creatures, we're often forced to constrain ourselves to fulfill our social roles. So it's understandable that our minds are sometimes overwhelmed.

Yoga has a real effect on this situation. In this book, I pass down several esoteric teachings of yoga practice.

Some of these yoga postures may look strange to you. Yoga involves diets and breathing methods that seem unusual. Most introductory books emphasize this strangeness and tell you that yoga is effective in some way, but do little to explain the essence or fundamentals of yoga.

I'm happy that yoga is becoming popular, but if teachers and students utilize only partial knowledge, problems can result. Yoga is truly yoga only when it's practiced both as a physical discipline for the mind and as mind training for the body. I want people to know more about yoga. Yoga has methods that can transform the human body and mind from deep within, creating effects that you may never have expected.

Yoga speaks only the truth

Yoga isn't a special teaching. It isn't meant to puzzle people with its mystery, or cause people to view it with absolute appreciation.

Yoga simply shows us the basis and conclusion and the truth and facts of our thoughts and behaviors. For example, yoga teaches us to be friendly to everyone – a basis of human life that even children know, but one that's also applicable to adults.

It also teaches us to love. This may be too abstract to understand with words alone, so let's put it this way: Do you prefer to love or hate others? Which feels better and more joyous?

Of course it's better to love than to hate. This is the basis and conclusion. Think of it this way: The lessons we learn in college are more difficult than those in kindergarten, but the fundamentals remain the same.

The same can be said about the body. *Asanas* are a collection of postures and movements that stabilize the body. The idea is that you feel comfortable, your mind calms down, and your body stays healthy by doing the movements. Zen means stability.

Yoga teaches that the best way to stabilize the body and mind is through breathing techniques, nutrition, and by using the body and mind itself. That's why I hope that this book will be read by many people, including athletes, scholars, people who are too busy with work to find time for exercise, and those who are engaged in a religious practice. Yoga is a collection of truths, and therefore doesn't conflict with any particular beliefs or thoughts.

Be grateful for illness

You may be thinking, "I'm not the way I should be. I want to be more vibrant." That's how I was before I started practicing yoga. Although we possess our mind and body, it's difficult to move them the way we'd like to.

Bad habits and customs left untreated can develop into sickness – but we can overcome them by training. You can train your body and mind to remember your natural state of being. The practice of yoga enables us to gain this sort of control over ourselves.

It's said that NASA, after researching numerous training methods of both East and West, adopted yoga as the most practical way to train its astronauts. That's because yoga contains the most profound understanding of the human body and mind.

In yoga, we believe that we can never be truly damaged by disease

– we can always stay healthy. Our life force serves to protect, sustain, and restore our health in a continuous cycle. Disease is simply a manifestation of our life force's attempt to protect our life.

On its own, life is very natural and balanced. Wild animals die, but not unnaturally as a result of disease, like humans. We get sick because our life force, which dislikes unnatural states of being, tries to restore balance. When you get sick, you should be grateful that your life force is warning you about the unnatural situation you're in.

Yoga is a way of training that we can practice in our daily lives to develop our ability to maintain balance. If you can understand balance in your mind and body, your life will be more joyful.

Spiritual trainings all over the world have origins in yoga. Lao Tzu, for example, taught a method for becoming empty. I-chin teaches *Yin* and *Yang*. The universe, nature, and human beings exist on a cycle that balances Yin and Yang. So in order to be healthy, we simply need to live as we are.

Buddha, Jesus, and Mohammad are said to have reached enlightenment by practicing yoga. Yoga originated in India about 5,000 years ago. But it wasn't established by just one person. Rather, it's a natural treatment, philosophy, and religion that people have developed based on their own experiences. Similar practices have been widely used in the Middle East and Asia. How could this be? Perhaps because there is only one truth of how we live and how we sustain our lives.

The fundamentals of other religions are the same as those of yoga.

For example, the Buddhist term *zen* is the equivalent of *antei*, or stability, in yoga. Likewise, *Shingon* means *toitsu*, or unification; *jodo* is *mushin*, or nonfixating mind; *hoge* means non-attachment; and *hokke* signifies offering prayer to everything. To be Christian is to believe in God's love. If you were to give Christianity a Buddhist-like name, it might be called the "Religion of God's Love." These ideas are found in yoga as well. This is the basic principle of the most natural, low-impact way to move one's physical body and one's mind/heart.

Why we need to learn about the spiritual world

It's said that this is an age of spirituality. That's because the scientific rationalism that created our modern society's abundance has developed a bad reputation. We now blame science for wars, inhumanity, and pollution.

I don't really agree with this. I think serious diseases require medicine and surgeries. Cars and airplanes have made things very convenient. We who use these things are the problem.

Humans need spirituality as well as science. There are things we can't really understand through science or philosophy. Nature and the universe are mysteries to us. Religion, or spirituality, is an acknowledgement of the unknown world. The age of spirituality occurs when science and spirituality coexist.

Einstein, when asked whether science could solve all the mysteries of the universe, responded, "It would be possible to describe everything scientifically, but it would make no sense; it would be without meaning, as if you described a Beethoven symphony as a variation of wave pressure."

When you want to know the truth, you need the ability both to think and to feel. However, having been raised with scientific rationalism, it's difficult for us to have a different point of view. So we begin with logical physical movements and a good diet to create a foundation, and then we meditate to develop our sensitivity and spiritual abilities.

In yoga, religion means to discover god within oneself. It is to see god in others and in nature. By doing so, you attain peace of mind for the first time.

Since I started practicing yoga, my lifestyle has become different from the average person's. Every day I meditate, read, and sleep a little. Forty years ago, I gave up all entertainments, because I didn't want to waste my time. I sleep a little whenever I want to, whether it's morning, afternoon, or night. I can stay awake as long as I want to if I try.

I consider everyone to be my children, brothers, or parents. My attitude never changes, whatever country I go to. I stopped writing journals and letters because I don't have anything to write. At one point, I didn't use the telephone for five years.

I lead my life this way because I've always wanted to know the truth. Humans can't possess two kinds of mind at once – love and hate, for example. In order to feel things correctly, you have to let go of them and observe them from a distance.

If you don't attain balance of mind, you can't reach the truth. You need to throw away everything that's unnecessary and attain a mind that doesn't get caught up. I'm not interested in things like status, honor, and money – just in seeking the truth. But I'm not saying everyone should be like me; I don't think they have to. I don't think there will be a time when everyone all around the world is awakened to the truth.

I just want you to know that there is a spiritual reality in this world. If you practice meditation, you will understand yourself and the world more profoundly and completely, from top to bottom. Though what I call truth is also a fact – the reality of human existence.

The ten steps to mastering yoga

Reading this, you may be thinking that yoga seems too difficult. But it's not. Yoga is actually very easy to understand because it teaches everything in order, from the start to the goal. Both the theories and practical methods are described in detail so that they fully penetrate your mind and body. All you have to do is add these ideas to your daily life.

By way of introduction, here's a simple example of a yoga pose in application: You sit down to take an exam, and your heart starts beating loud and fast as the exam is distributed. You nervousness increases as you try to calm yourself down. What would you do in this situation?

First, stretch your arms perpendicular to your sides, bending your elbows 90 degrees and making fists with your hands. Take a deep breath. Slowly exhale and bring your head down as you push on your solar plexus with your fingertips.

You should feel calm now. When you're nervous, your shoulders are stiff and your chest is tight. By stimulating the appropriate parts of your body with breath and movement, you create a calm state, physically and biologically. You build confidence inside your body.

When you lower your head, you feel calm. In Islam, when people pray to Allah they sit on the ground and stretch out their arms with their forehead on the ground. It's the same principle. You can take a deep breath by stretching your arms up high. You can do abdominal breathing, which calms you down, by lowering your head and stretching your arms forward. Doing breathing techniques and poses in the movements of the prayer calms you down.

If your shoulders are stiff right now, do this: As in the previous exercise, bend your elbows 90 degrees and as you breathe in, open your chest so that your shoulder blades come together. Hold your breath and energize your entire body, then drop your hands suddenly and exhale. If you do this about three times, your shoulders will feel better immediately.

This is the beginning of yoga practice. Yoga describes the path to liberating the mind and body and realizing a natural way of being in ten steps. These steps form a natural process in the practice of yoga, and are very efficient. I'll describe them in more detail later, but I'd like to introduce them here very briefly.

1. *Yama and Niyama:* The study of the two different kinds of mind: the one you should have and the one you shouldn't have. But it's not just preaching – it's preparing the mind to begin yoga.
2. *Asanas:* A way of training from outside the body, using active and inactive poses. More a physical than a mental preparation.
3. *Pranayama:* A way of training from within the body. Here we discuss breathing techniques, diet, and ways of studying.
4. *Pratyahara:* A method for controlling oneself biologically and mentally at will.

These first four steps encompass the practice known as *hatha* yoga, designed to create a natural mind and body. From the fifth step on, the practice is known as raja yoga, primarily a meditation practice.

5. *Dharana:* Nature balances itself through repeating changes, harmony, and stability. When we fight this natural balance, problems occur in our mind and body. This step is the practice of harmonizing the mind, body, lifestyle, and environment. It cultivates *tanden* power, the ability to concentrate, and consciousness.
6. *Dhyana:* This practice enables you to achieve a state of total relaxation of mind and body, through the physical practice of complete nonattachment.
7. *Bhakti:* A practice to empty the mind, *bhakti* is different from ordinary worship. It's also called "worshipping practice of the mind."

Up to this seventh step, yoga practice is about developing the self, regaining the self that's been affected by society. From the eighth step on, it is a training to achieve self-enlightenment and a practice to expand your potential.

8. *Samadhi:* Oneself and others become one, harmonizing and cooperating to sustain each other.
9. *Buddhi:* A practice to achieve Buddha-mind, which honors all people and nature.
10. *Prasada:* A practice to experience true joy with the mind and body.

Physical and mental training should be done at the same time

As we've seen, yoga can be categorized briefly into two groups: *hatha* yoga and *raja* yoga.

In hatha yoga, we discuss physical education, such as sports and martial arts. In raja yoga we discuss intellectual education, the search for philosophical truth, and moral education, the search for spiritual enlightenment. In this way, yoga covers all three areas: physical, intellectual, and spiritual enlightenment.

I stated previously that the spread of "false yoga" has become a problem. It's false because it teaches only the hatha part of yoga. It's like the circus or wrestling. People train their bodies to do things that are useless. It's merely a partial training, in what should be a holistic practice.

Yoga is sacred – its purpose is to search for something beneficial to you and to others as well. But false yoga is worldly, taking only one's own profits and benefits into account.

Think about practicing hatha yoga in a raja yoga way, and raja yoga in a hatha yoga way – for example, training your mind while you do postures. Understand that yoga practice is not physical training for the body, but physical training for the mind

For the purposes of this book, I've organized the ten steps into four chapters. Yoga training consists of different types of practices, with different characteristics. Some require detailed description and some need to be practiced firsthand in order to be understood. Let's begin with the first step of yoga, training the mind – which ultimately is the conclusion as well.

The first step: The Spiritual Path – Yama and Niyama

Yama refers to prohibitions, or things you must not do. *Niyama,* on the other hand, refers to things you should do and are encouraged to do.

The *Yamas* are as follows:

1. *Do not kill, harm, offend, hurt, or persecute.* This teaching instructs you think of a way to support all life forms including yourself, friends, animals, plants, and the environment. Nature is precious. Humans don't have the right to destroy it.

2. *Do not speak or act dishonestly.* You should be able to say "right" when something is right, "wrong" when it's wrong, or "I don't

know." It may seem like a small thing, but there are many times when it takes a lot of courage just to speak your mind. It's difficult to live without lying to yourself, but it's the only true way to live. I live in a way that's true to myself. I'm a man, so I think like a man, and perform my responsibilities and duties like a man. I'm sixty years old, so I live like I'm sixty years old. It's about being honest and living life as it really is.

3. *Do not steal.* This doesn't just mean "don't steal things." It also means that you shouldn't speak about things you've heard or read in books as if you really know them, without having experienced them yourself. Even a criminal feels guilty when he steals things or money, but people rarely feel guilty when they steal someone's opinion or philosophy. If you agree with another's opinion or thought, then make it your own. But in order to do so, you need to really feel it through your own life experiences. It's like driving a care – even if you read a lot of books about the mechanics of cars or that explain how to drive, you can't actually drive until you do it yourself. This isn't just a problem for individuals – it's also a problem of societies and nations. For example, I believe that much of the materialistic culture of modern Japan is based on stealing what Westerners have spent much effort to create. But we rarely acknowledge this fact. Rather, we go about pretending that we built these things entirely on our own. There's no feeling of either gratitude or guilt. There's no fraction of regret or creativity. "Do not steal" is a criticism of attitudes like this.

4. *Do not possess evil desires.* Receive only that which should naturally be given to you. This is not an evil desire, but a natural desire. But humans too often desire things they're less likely to be given. We think we should be praised, get a raise, or be better understood. And we think such desires are natural. But to me these are evil desires. You think that what you have is yours, and that what others have is yours too. You're looking for pennies from heaven. This creates dissatisfaction, complaint, anxiety, hatred, and anger. But in the end, problems turn out the way they should. You should accept destiny. Even if it's difficult, look at suffering as a valuable opportunity, and use that energy to live in a way that's true to yourself. In short, allow yourself to enter a state of surrender.

5. *Do not possess.* Not possessing means having only the necessities and things that are given to you naturally. I'll expand upon this. Think of everything as public. Rather than "my land," think of land as belonging to all of society. Every living thing has a right to utilize

the planet earth. Humans, grasses, trees, dogs, and cats all have the same right. Humans have a duty to use the planet in a way that benefits every living thing.

The *Niyamas* are as follows:

1. *Purify your mind and body.* Your mind and body become impure when you're not true to yourself. For example, if I eat things that suit my body, the blood I produce will be suitable for me. However, if I eat something that doesn't suit my body, the blood I create will be unsuitable. Unsuitable blood is thick and dirty, and causes disease. If you're true to yourself, your body and mind are pure. It's about finding out what it's like to be "yourself." In short, you shouldn't live pretending and being dishonest to yourself. Humans are easily influenced. If you really want to quit smoking, for example, you shouldn't forget to discard the matches, lighter, cigarette case, and ashtray along with the cigarettes. It's important to eliminate things that cause struggles.

2. *Be satisfied.* Learn to be fulfilled. The universe and nature give humans just what they need. When you get sick, be sick. What you're given at any one moment is what you most need at that moment, what is most valuable. For example, my right hand, which is writing just now, was given by nature, and nothing is lacking or extraneous. I wouldn't be better off if my fingers could bend outward, or if my wrists rotated 360 degrees. And what if something were added? Even if it weighed only a few ounces, it would be annoying. I am allowed to posses this right hand, which is a gift from nature.

3. *Have boundaries.* Separate what you know and what you don't. In order to understand the truth, you have to look at things without illusion or misunderstanding. When you study, you have to organize your brain; otherwise, you will feel unnecessarily anxious and your brain won't function. Having boundaries is also about being unaffected by your emotions – happiness, anger, sadness, or joy.

4. *Be disciplined.* In order to live in this modern, civilized, social world, we need discipline. Humans have a greater mental capacity than other animals do. Animals are exposed to nature. We, on the other hand, use our mental abilities to protect our minds and bodies from nature, and to spoil ourselves. We need to consciously train ourselves to adapt to our surroundings. The more advanced our civilization is, the more training we need. And not just physical

training – there are other important methods we can use, such as reading. Reading good books, taking in knowledge, does much to nourish the spirit. I'm always feeding my mind with new knowledge, and try to read at least three books a day. But only you can determine what books are most suitable for you.

5. *Pray to god.* In yoga, god is not a being particular to any one religion or religious sect. God is about discovering preciousness in all matter. Let's take our feet, for example. Feet are only feet if you think that's what they are. The moment you come to think of them as god, that's religion. Most religions worship god, pray to god, ask god for things. But in yoga, god is different – god always exists right here, in you and in me. Only you can save yourself

Yoga makes us happy. That's because yoga ties everything to our true nature. The virtues and truths that we seek – be they health, beauty, enlightenment, happiness, peace, freedom, joy, stability, or harmony – are all different terms for our nature. Suffering, on the other hand, is both the result of an unnatural state and at the same time the process whereby we return to our natural state.

Yoga's most important purpose is to awaken people to the idea that god is within them and to help them understand the law of karma. The god within is nature within, which I teach as *seimei-soku-shin,* literally, "(what) the life force is doing is what god is doing. Your life force is god, therefore you are god. Your life is god and nature.

Karma teaches you that you have created your own worries and that you alone can solve them. You can control your own destiny, health and disease, enlightenment and confusion, and happiness and unhappiness. You have the key.

Yoga teaches you how to use that key. Its specific techniques teach you how to apply the law of nature.

What's the key to being at one with nature? Maintaining balance and stability through change. Imbalance and strain force the mind and body into unnatural states. Being aware of your habits, customs, conditioning, biases, addictions, excesses, and irrelevance is critical to maintaining balance.

The practice and philosophy of yoga teaches you to avoid and eliminate what's unnatural, and maintain and recover what's natural.

I will now introduce you to the second step of yoga – *asanas* – as well as inactive poses and *zaho.*

Chapter 1

The Secret of Body and Mind

Even our feet have minds of their own

If someone has a stomach problem, it is reflected in their body constitution.

When someone comes to me complaining of physical or mental discomfort, I can tell where the problem is by looking at them. People often ask me how I'm able to detect, diagnose, and cure disease. They think it's mysterious, but really it's quite simple.

You can see what the problem is by looking at the body. People with stomach problems always have a certain way of breathing, and their body is distorted to compensate. If you know where the trouble is, all you need to do is correct their body and their breathing to bring them closer to a natural state and solve the problem.

When I treat a disease, I think about the body's fundamentals – the spine and muscles. If these are normal you're healthy, but if they're abnormal you're unhealthy. If that's the case, you need certain practices to get back to your proper natural state.

As we go through our normal activities, our spine and muscles are constantly being tilted and distorted. If this is fixed right away it won't cause serious problems, but if it becomes a habit, it can cause disease.

So what can we do to maintain our body's natural health? The second step of yoga, asanas, is a training method based on the study of the entire mind-body system, called *migamae,* or preparing the body. The first step is *kokorogamae,* preparing the mind.

There's no need for difficult postures

The second step is training the body from the outside, through inactive postures such as Cat Pose, headstand, and meditation, and active postures, which will be discussed in chapter 3.

These postures not only correct tilted and distorted alignment, they also help you discover which areas of the body are problematic. Because the postures are all designed to suit the body naturally, any difficulty practicing them may indicate an area of weakness in the body.

Yoga teaches us to move rationally and economically through our daily life. But what's ideal is different for each person, just as everyone's body type and constitution is different. When you stand, you won't be stable unless you find the correct stance for your specific frame and constitution. I need to sit with my legs open in a certain way that suits me, or I can't find a stable posture.

Instability strains our body and mind. In our body, this strain manifests as pain, tiredness, numbness, and other sensations. But don't think of these symptoms as negative. Rather, accept them as a warning from the life force or divinity within you. Without these symptoms, your body would get even worse, and eventually more serious symptoms would appear.

The same thing can be said about the mind. Unnatural ways of thinking and feeling cause worry. These worries, too, are a warning that you're doing something wrong.

In yoga, nobody should tell you that you absolutely have to do difficult postures. It's up to you whether you want to do extreme postures. Because each posture is made up of different steps, when you're beginning you can easily do just the steps that don't strain your body – the ones that make your body happy. Eventually, you'll be able to do difficult postures relatively easily, and you may want to learn them.

Doing yoga is similar to the physical training one does for sports or martial arts, but the meaning is very different. Training for sports or martial arts makes your body like a superman's, but it doesn't acknowledge the mind. Yoga not only makes your body strong, it also makes your mind calm and peaceful – and enables you to move very quickly and promptly.

That's because yoga enhances your ability to relax, to be calm, and to let go of unnecessary tension, and creates in you the readiness to cope with any situation. It gives you the ability to balance in any position, because it trains you in every posture known to man.

Sexual drive makes your blood acidic

Before I introduce the postures, I'd like to explore the secret of the body-mind structure.

We conduct a variety of movements in our lives. Whether these movements are conscious or subconscious, they influence us in some way without our knowing it.

No other animal makes as many conscious movements as humans do. However, there are really only twelve basic movements:

1. Bend forward
2. Bend back
3. Tilt to the left
4. Tilt to the right
5. Twist to the left
6. Twist to the right
7. Li ft the center
8. Lower the center
9. Tighten
10. Relax
11. Stretch, or expand
12. Contract

The autonomic nervous system helps to govern the body's subconscious functions, such as the activities of the heart and stomach. Within this system, the sympathetic nerves stimulate functioning, and the parasympathetic nerves suppress functioning.

Another subconscious element is the body fluid. In a normal state, human blood is slightly alkaline, but it can become overly acidic or alkaline when one eats, exercises, breathes, or takes part in other activities. It changes constantly throughout the day.

Let's put these conscious behaviors and subconscious body functions together and categorize them in order to understand how they relate:

1. Stimulation of the sympathetic nerves makes the blood acidic. This results from moving the spine, bending forward, exercising, thinking, sexual drive or appetite, bathing, anger, hatred, or eating meat and acidic foods.
2. Stimulation of the parasympathetic nerves makes the blood alkaline. This results from moving the abdomen, bending backward, meditating, deep breathing, warm baths, sleeping, laughing, enjoying, being happy, or eating vegetarian and alkalizing foods.

A forceful abdomen leads to good health

In yoga, it's considered important to move with your whole being in a natural state. The center point – which is used to move the mind and

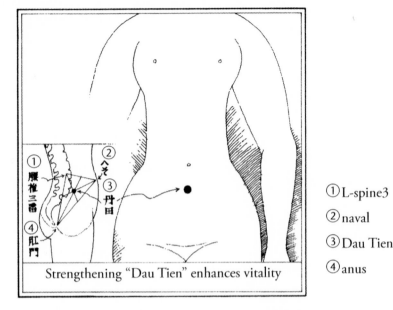

① 腰椎三番
② へそ
③ 丹田
④ 肛門

① L-spine3
② naval
③ Dau Tien
④ anus

Strengthening "Dau Tien" enhances vitality

body in an integrated, holistic way – is called *uddiyana* in yoga, *tanden* (tan tien) in Chinese, and hara in Japanese. Physically, it's your lower back and abdomen.

If you enhance the operation of this center point, your life force energy and your ability to sustain health will increase. To create tanden is one of the most important achievements in yoga training. Tanden is one of the most important beliefs in yoga; that's why it's called uddiyana, or throne of god. When I explain this concept to foreigners, I refer to it as a holy center.

Strong tanden enhances the life force

To enhance your tanden power, try to tighten your sphincter muscles. Relax your upper body (*Kyo,* or empty) and bring your force to the lower body (*Jitsu,* or solid). In Japan, since ancient time, we have said, *Jokyo-Kajittus* (empty top and solid bottom) or *Zukan-Sokunetsu* (cold head and warm feet, in other words, cool the head but warm the feet).

When someone needs to calm down physically and emotionally, we tell them to lower their hips, bring force to the inner knees and big toes, straighten the neck, open the chest, and breathe deeply. This helps bring energy to tanden.

Keep this in mind at all times, not just when you're practicing yoga.

How to move the head and eyes

Let's look at other details of body structure that can be used to diagnose physical conditions.

When we're trying to remember something, we lean our head back. While we do so subconsciously, biologically speaking it actually stimulates the memory storage area in the cerebrum. When we're contemplating something, we lean our head forward, like Rodin's *The Thinker,* because it activates the function of the cerebral cortex, particularly the frontal lobe. When the head is tilted to the side, it stimulates harmonization of the cerebral cortex and memory storage; we do this when we're organizing thoughts based on our own ideas. Therefore, in yoga, the posture that enhances memory involves leaning your head back.

The same is true for the eyes. If you do these movements with a strong intent, you can stimulate or calm the body:

- Moving the eyeballs to the center stimulates the spinal cord.
- Moving the eyeballs upward stimulates the brain.
- Moving the eyeballs down stimulates the abdominal area.
- Moving the eyeballs away from each other alkalizes and calm your mind.
- Moving the eyeballs to the center makes your body acidic and excited or nervous.

When your eyes aren't balanced, it's a sign that there's a problem in your internal organs.

- If your pupils are on the upper part of your eyes, your blood's components are imbalanced, causing an imbalance in your body.
- If one pupil is lower than the other, the organs on that side of the body are lowered as well. If it's on the left, you have stomach problems; on the right, liver problems.

The eyes are closely related to the entire body, so be aware of the position of your eyes when you do yoga postures.

As you move your body, there are a few basic principles for moving the eyes. These natural movements will help prevent stress or strain on your body or mind.

- When you arch your back, look up.
- When you bend forward, look down.
- When you twist your body, look in the same direction as the twist.

Many people have eye problems such as nearsightedness and astigmatism. While these problems may be caused by reading books on the train or by working all day at a desk, in some cases mental issues materialize as disease. You become nearsighted not because you can't see things, but because you don't want to see them. And as your eyes develop bad habits, your vision gets worse.

Eyes are strong organs that don't wear out no matter how much we use them; we all use our eyes for sixteen or seventeen hours straight, every day. So if you have a problem, do eye exercises. Open your eyes wide and roll them. Look at something far in the distance, then look at something closer, and keep repeating. This can improve your sight.

You can tell the disease by looking at the fingers

The nerves of the internal organs and muscles are connected to the brain, which controls them, but the peripheral nerves are spread throughout the body. In yoga these are called charkas, and in oriental medicine they're known as acupuncture points. Acupuncture points can exist in unexpected places; for example, the points for the sexual organs are on the palms.

The movements of the hands are deeply connected to the brain. The reason that the human cerebrum is more developed than that of other animals – so much so that we're able to speak languages – is because we have hands that we can move in many ways. When you tighten your hands, your brain contracts.

The spinal nerves from cervical vertebra ④ to thoracic vertebra ② connect to the hands, and are therefore closely related to all the internal organs. In addition, the sympathetic nerves of the autonomic nervous system run to the pinkies, and the vagus nerves run to the thumbs. The strength of the palms is related to the ribs, as well as to the throat, eyes, ears, nose, small intestines, and sexual organs. Each finger has a different nerve that reflects differently on the internal organs.

You can check the condition of your body by looking at your hands. Let's experiment. Stretch your arms out parallel to the floor with the palms facing down.

1. If your wrists are tilted toward your thumbs, with your middle fingers at the center, your body is acidic.
2. If your wrists are tilted toward your pinkies, your body is alkaline.

The health of your internal organs can be determined by looking at your hand. If your fingers are all nice and straight naturally, you're healthy, but if they're bent it means the organ that's connected to that particular finger is always tense and tired.

Here's a way to test if your liver is weak. Keep your pinky, ring finger, and middle finger straight together, and separate them from the index finger. If the fingers tend to separate as you open your index finger, your liver is tired.

Let's take a deeper look at how our fingers reflect our body and mind.

- **Thumb:** The thumb is connected to the parasympathetic nerves, and relates to the components and condition of the blood. It's connected to the brain, which means you can calm yourself down by rubbing the bottom of the thumb. It's also connected to the speech center, so you can correct stutters and speech defects by stimulating it. Massaging the area between the bottom of the thumb and the index finger stimulates the intestines and liver, improving elimination. The thumb is also related to cervical vertebra #4.

- **Index finger:** The index finger relates to the liver, stomach, intestine, spleen, and pancreas. The right index finger relates to the liver; the left to the stomach. If you touch your left index finger when you've overeaten, it will feel hard.

- **Middle finger:** The middle finger relates to the circulatory system, including the heart, kidneys, and blood vessels. If your heart suddenly feels abnormal, press the point at the center of your palm directly below the left middle finger. It also relates to the spine, so energy tends to stay in this finger. If you relax the other fingers and do *gassho* (prayer *mudra*) or mudra (two fingers touching, see Lotus Pose, page 60), your mind and body will calm down.

- **Ring finger:** The ring finger relates to the nervous system. It's particularly deeply connected to the central optic nerve. The ring fingers of some epileptic or deaf people don't move. It also relates to the weak points of the human body below the solar plexus to the navel; so if you hold the ring finger, you'll feel more active. We call this the medicine finger in Japanese because it relates to your life force energy.

- **Pinky:** The pinky relates to the sexual organ, lungs, and sympathetic nerves. A person whose pinky is usually bent tends to be frustrated and angry. If you can't straighten your pinky, the rib or vertebrae on that side may have a problem.

In the yoga *dojo,* we practice touching and rotating each finger as a morning routine. If any one of them is hard to move or swollen, we continue to work on it by rotating and rubbing it. If you do this exercise in the morning, while your nerves are more sensitive, your body will feel warmer. Because the fingers are connected to different body parts, you can fix various problems by stimulating the fingers. Or if you want to you're your head, relax your hands.

If you take care of your feet, you won't get sick

The nerves leading from the lumbar region and sacrum are in the feet. So the condition of the feet is related to that of the sexual organs, urinary tract, and cerebrum. In addition, most of the blood that travels through our body goes to the feet. The blood travels down easily, thanks to gravity, but since the feet are so far from the heart, traveling up is more of a strain. That's why aging in the feet leads to aging in the entire body.

Feet serve as tools for walking, as a foundation to support the body, as the controller of blood circulation – and they relate to every organ at once.

For example, the right foot influences the circulation of blood to the lungs and veins. If you break or sprain your right foot and it remains weak, you could easily develop lung problems. The left foot has to do with the arteries, so if it's weak you're even more likely to have a lung problem.

The inner thigh muscle relates to the sex organs and urinary tract. Children with *enuresis* (bed-wetting) can improve the problem by stretching their inner thighs. When the Achilles tendon is contracted, one's weight is drawn backward. This decreases the strength of the pelvis and the abdomen accordingly, resulting in the lowering of the internal organs, menstruation problems because the blood circulation is enhanced.

When the calves are tight, the stomach and intestines, as well as the sexual function, become weak. If your heels are flat rather than round, it means that your weight tends to be on your heels. This raises the pelvis, drains energy from the lower hip and abdomen, and expands the skull, slowing you down and making you dull-witted and bored.

Like the fingers, each toe relates to certain parts of your body. The backs of your feet relate to the entire body. If any part of the foot is abnormal – bent or tight, for example – the internal organs that are related to that part get sick, too. So any abnormality in an organ will manifest in the feet and signify a problem.

Let's take a look at each toe.

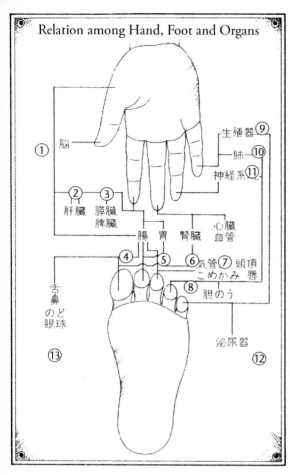

Relation among Hand, Foot and Organs

① brain
③ liver
③ spleen
④ intestine
⑤ stomach
⑥ kidney
⑦ heart blood vessel
⑧ bronchium
temple
lips
gall bladder
⑨ reproductive organs
⑩ lung
⑪ nervous system
⑫ urinary organ
⑬ tongue
nose
throat
eyeball

- *The first toe (big toe):* The first toe relates to the parasympathetic nerves and controls body fluid. It also relates to the kidneys, throat, tongue, nose, eyes, and intestines. If your first toe is plump, you may be overeating or suffering from high blood pressure, diabetes, hypertrophic liver, or *empyema.* Holding a yoga posture in which this toe is tightened fills your abdominal area with force, helping you use your body without excess strain or exhaustion.
- *The second toe:* The second toe relates to the digestive system.
- *The third toe:* The third toe relates to the circulatory system and intestines, as well as to the bronchi, lips, temples, and vertex. If your second or third toe is tense, you may have problems with your stomach. If it's swollen, you may suffer from hyperacidity or overeating.
- *The fourth toe:* The fourth toe relates to the nerves, gallbladder, and

lungs. If it's weak and lifted, you're more likely to get tuberculosis. If it's stiff, inflexible, and lifted, your bile is not being secreted effectively, or you may be gassy or constipated.

- *The fifth toe:* The fifth toe relates to the sympathetic nerves, urinary tract, and sex organs. It also relates to the ability to tighten the sphincter, so massaging it can help heal hemorrhoids. If it's stiff and bent down, your internal organs may be low (*splanchnoptosis*) or your uterus may be located in the wrong place.

You can correct certain physical problems by moving your toes like fingers. Your toes are usually tight and confined inside shoes. It's good to pull, bend, and rotate each toe occasionally. That's especially important with stiff, cold, and unusual toes. Treating your toes is very simple but can be surprisingly effective. Just like the saying "rolling stones gather no moss," if you move your toes around frequently, you won't get athlete's foot.

Let's look at rest of the leg. The knees relate to lumbar vertebra #3, which controls blood circulation and is in direct proportion to the strength of your tanden. Achilles tendons relate to the blood flow in the brain.

The thighs relate to lumbar vertebrae #1 and #2, and demonstrate the nutritional status of the entire body. The outer thighs are connected to the intestines and lower back. If this area is stiff, your lower back is strained. The inner things relate to the elimination process of the urinary tract and the sex organs.

Correcting the way your legs move is very important. Because leg movements are the widest and largest body movements, they're the most difficult aspect of the postures I'll be introducing, but for the same reason they can be quite effective.

So what about movements that utilize the head, hands, legs, and the rest of the body?

The healthy way to stand, sit, and walk

You can rest your muscles by stretching them. If you move your body for work or sport, your muscles contract and need rest. If you leave them contracted, they'll become stiff. After you exercise, try to do something that feels good – that corrects your pulse, eases your breath, and makes your body light. If you move on the out-breath, communicate with your body, and let your mind smile while you use your body, you won't hurt your muscles. Begin by thinking about sitting movements.

When we sit calmly, we separate our knees. When we're nervous, our knees are tight and our hands, shoulders, and neck are stiff. People often say "relax your shoulders" to calm someone down, but you also need to stabilize your brain by letting go of tension in the hands, shoulders, and neck.

You can relax your body by holding your palms face up, which stimulates the parasympathetic nerves. When the palms face down, the sympathetic nerves are stimulated, which tenses the body.

When you sit with your palms face down on your thighs, you look formal; with your palms face up, you look more relaxed.

When you sit for a long time, your body contracts. When this happens, it's a good idea to stand up and shake your body, relaxing the muscles, enhancing blood flow along the spine, and calming your mind. This is the same mechanism that helps children fall asleep when you sing them a lullaby and rock them. When your body stays in the same posture for too long, the spine doesn't get enough blood and the muscles become stiff. Shaking your body helps you relax and maintains your health.

The way you sit is a reflection of your body and mind. Some of these examples may be relevant to your situation.

1. If one leg is higher than the other when you sit, it means that the internal organs on that side are weak. If it's the right leg that's affected, it means that the liver is weak; if it's the left, the stomach. Unconsciously, you are performing an action to relax it into balance.
2. If your legs are restless, your pelvic bones may be twisted or you may suffer from nervousness.
3. When you sit on the floor with your legs to one side, you're most likely to place your legs to the side opposite the side that's abnormally contracted. Everyone does this without thinking. Having this information enables you to correct the distorted posture.
4. If you sit with your hips very low, you may have problems with your abdomen or urinary tract.
5. If, when you sit with your legs wide open, your back is rounded and your pubic bone sticks out, you may sometimes have problems completing your elimination.

If you have a job that requires a lot of sitting – one that uses the brain and hands – you will subconsciously choose a posture that concentrates energy in the lower body. When you sit for long periods of time, you don't exercise your legs, blood congests around the abdomen, the organs lose their ability to contract, and the heart becomes weak. Moreover, the organs move lower, and excess blood in the abdominal area and tiredness in the brain create an occupational disease. To prevent this, rub and move your legs and abdomen often to stimulate blood flow.

When you sit in *seiza*, a seated position with your legs crossed, your legs become numb because blood flow to the legs and internal organs is constricted, and the Achilles tendons are contracted. If you're going to spend some time sitting in *seiza*, stretch your Achilles tendons beforehand. This will enhance blood flow and prevent numbness. If blood circulates properly to the internal organs, numbness won't occur.

So how should we stand and walk?

You should stand with your legs hip-width apart, concentrating the weight in the arch of the foot. And you should walk using the entire sole of the foot.

If the pace of your legs doesn't match, there may be problem in your internal organs. If you walk with eyes closed and tend to the right, you can improve your organs by making your right footstep larger intentionally.

The best walking pace is one in which you can breathe most easily (that doesn't necessarily mean walking slowly). Lift your chest, tighten your abdomen, tuck your chin, pull your shoulder blades together, straighten your neck, and release the tension in your shoulders. Your brain will stay stable and your mind will be clear.

Whenever you use one part of your body, try to relax the other side. If you're using your right hand, relax your left hand, and if you are using right leg, relax your left leg. This prevents you from feeling tired and helps you recover from fatigue.

When you tighten both sides, your force is divided and you can't use your full strength. In short, it's best to do something that focuses your entire body. That's the natural way.

You might also want to try doing things opposite the way you normally do them. If you tend to look down, try arching your back.

In yoga, we practice walking backwards like children. This helps keep your back straight, and you can walk beautifully.

Self-check based on your sleeping posture

Watching someone sleep tells you about their health. Check yourself by looking at how you sleep.

1. *Face down:* If you sleep on your belly, your liver and chest area may be suppressed or low. This position is an indication of insufficient elimination or respiratory function. And because it strains the

hip, your sexual hormones may be out of balance, resulting in low sex drive.

2. *On your side:* You can determine the problem by looking at which side is up. People usually sleep with the side that's exhausted pointing up so that the problematic parts can rest. Because your temperature rises on the side that faces down, having the affected side up keeps it cool and rests it.

If you have liver problem, you'll tend to sleep with your right side up; if you have spleen or stomach problems, you'll sleep with your left side up to protect those organs. But if the fatigue builds up to the point of chronic stiffness, you'll sleep with the bad side down to increase blood flow into the area to warm it.

If you sleep on your side with both legs bent, you may have problems with your digestive system. If you sleep on your side with one leg bent, you may have problems you're your urinary tract.

3. *Face up:* The healthiest option is to sleep on your back with your arms and legs straight, as in the Corpse Pose *(Savasana)*. This sleeping posture eliminates stress and tiredness. If you're severely exhausted, sleep with your knees up in order to relax lumbar vertebra #1. This also relaxes your head.

If you have trouble sleeping with your legs outstretched, you have an underlying problem somewhere. For example, if you cross your legs or bend your knees, you likely have skin problems such as pimples, freckles, or athlete's foot because your pubic bones are off, as well as imperfect elimination, resulting in constipation.

When you cross your legs, the internal organs on the same side as the leg that's on top may be weak. If the right leg is on top, you may have liver problem; if the left, stomach problems.

If you spread your legs wide, you may have problems with your large intestines or sex organs.

If you bend your knees inward, your digestive system may be weak.

If you bend one knee and put it on top of the other knee, you may have problem with your sex organs and urinary tract.

4. *Hands up:* This indicates problems with overeating. You're trying to relax your stomach by spreading your ribs.

5. *Lowering a shoulder or contracting a leg:* If you lower your right shoulder or contract your right leg as you sleep, you may have problems with your right abdominal area or hip.

6. *Pillowing your head on your arm:* Using a pillow distorts the body, so it's better to go without. If you sleep with your hands interlaced under your head, it indicates that your shoulders and neck are stiff and your head is tired. If you can't sleep without a pillow, you may be humpbacked and your neck may be contracted.

7. *Moving up or down:* If you tend to move up toward the top of the bed as you sleep, you probably have very good blood circulation, which makes you feel hot. If you tend to move down toward the bottom of the bed, your blood circulation is poor, making you feel cold. You may be lacking vitamins and minerals, and may have nerve problems.

8. Hands on your chest: This may indicate psychological problems. Because your heart is like a pump, you can slow it down by putting your hands on it. This posture suggests that you may be having nightmares.

Your state of mind can cause disease

The mind influences the body, and the body influences the mind. Your feet and hands also have minds of their own, in a sense. When you're happy your hands and feet are warm, and when you're afraid or worried your hands and feet are cold. When you feel safe, you stand strong, with your feet apart, but when you're afraid your legs are tight together, lacking energy. If your legs are stiff and tired due to lack of exercise, you don't feel well.

This happens not just in your hands and feet but everywhere in your body.

Bad posture can also cause a troubled mind. As proof, if you correct your bad posture, you'll feel good.

If you're slow to move or to make decisions, you can practice postures that arch your back such as Bow Pose (p.44), or jump rope to become quicker. Your lower back and first toes determine your quickness. If your lower back is stiff and inflexible, your movements and brain function will tend to be slow.

Emotions and biological desires are both expressions of normal physical needs, so you can't suppress or eliminate them. If you do, abnormal stimuli will build up inside you, possibly resulting in abnormal postures or movements.

If you want to heal your body, you need to take care of your body and your mind. The same is true for healing your mind. I'd like to introduce sixteen basic silent postures that help balance an abnormal body and mind.

MAINTAINING YOUR HEALTH WITH SILENT POSTURES

Postures to beautify your body

We should try to maintain a correct posture at all times. Correct posture leads to correcting and enhancing your entire physiology and psychology. In yoga, we call this *Iigi-Soku-Buppo,* meaning that to live according to the righteous disciplines and rules that define life in a Zen Buddhist temple is the premise of learning Buddhism, and also that this premise itself is Buddhism.

Bad posture – for example, hunching your upper body for long periods of time at work – creates pressure in your stomach and lungs. Your breath becomes short and shallow, and your shoulders and neck become stiff, resulting in bad blood circulation to your brain. You get tired both physically and mentally. Even if you do hunch forward, if you stretch out your chest and breathe deeply you can still have good posture.

Fatigue or sickness of the mind and body is caused by distortion of the muscles and spine due to the prolonged holding of unnatural postures. If you eliminate the unnatural, you can keep your body and mind healthy and beautiful.

I'd like to introduce some of the silent yoga postures. As they are very basic, I'd like you to master them all, even if you don't have a physical or mental problem. The effects of these postures are countless: you can improve your physical strength, discover or prevent any disease, or tone your body beautifully. These are good to practice for a period of time every morning just after you wake up.

Some of these postures may be difficult for beginners, so before we proceed let's practice some body-building exercises that don't require any equipment.

Body-building exercises that don't use equipment

This very simple yoga-like exercise is similar to image training. People often make excuses for not exercising because they don't have the space or time, or they're not well physically. But being inactive can cause your muscles to degenerate. Even if you're busy you can practice this method anytime, anywhere. Here's what to do:

Tighten the muscles that you intend to exercise as if you're carrying something. Do this throughout your body. The key is to breathe with force.

For instance, lower your hips, tighten your arms as if you're holding a heavy rock, and straighten your hips and arms as if lifting the rock to eye level. You can exercise your entire body in creative ways: pretend to release an arrow from a bow, or act like you're shot-putting or pulling on a chest expander or elastic exercise band. Five to ten minutes of this should be enough.

It may look ridiculous but it's actually very logical. We can develop our muscles through very simple, regular exercise every day. If you hold your breath and tense your body for six to ten seconds once a day, you can develop your muscles very quickly.

This training method is very useful not only for those who want to maintain their health, but also for those who are sick in bed. If you have a problem in your abdominal area, you can exercise your hands, feet, and neck. Even exercising a finger can help, because the body's muscles are all related to each other and work together.

Use caution before practicing any posture

The purpose of the mental and physical training of yoga is to reach nirvana. In other words, its aim is the absolute liberation of mind, body, and life.

The goal of sports is generally to develop the body, but yoga's goal is to control oneself by harmonizing body and mind. So don't forget to focus and calm your mind in addition to balancing your breath.

Practice each posture front, back, left, and right. For example, if you lie down facing up, follow it by lying face down; if you bend forward, bend backward next in order to create balance.

Here are some other rules I'd like you to follow:

1. Go to the bathroom before you practice. Exercising with a full bladder or bowel can be harmful. And always wait at least one hour after a meal or after consuming alcohol before practicing.
2. Relax your body and mind before you practice. Relax your body by stretching, and your mind by *gassho* (holding your palms together in front of your chest in prayer position) or by laughing. For both, deep breath and *zazen* (sitting meditation) are good.
3. Enjoy your practice. If you practice unwillingly, your body will become tense and your center will become unstable.

4. Practice with no thoughts. Don't think, and practice as your body moves naturally.

5. Focus on the rhythm of your breath. In principle, when doing postures you should move during the out-breath. When you breathe out, your body is looser and not as likely to become strained, so your inner ability is enhanced.

6. Move slowly. Don't move your body by bouncing.

7. Visualize your movements and postures clearly in your head as you do them. Before you do a posture, focus your awareness on your tanden and gradually move it to the body parts you're trying to work.

8. As you finish each posture, relax for a second. Doing a posture creates extreme tension, so follow each posture with the Corpse Pose (exercise 1, below) and wait for your breath to calm down before you move on to the next one.

Now try the following postures one by one. Even if you can't do them all, don't try so hard that you strain yourself. As the days go by, you'll come to do them naturally.

1. Corpse Pose (Savasana)

For recovery. Practice this between postures for increased effectiveness.

This posture helps you recover from fatigue. Practice it as a short break following the other postures, which I'll introduce later, in a relaxed manner, as if lying on the mighty ocean. Practicing Corpse Pose makes your previous postures even more effective, because it is in this posture that the stimulation from the previous posture is assimilated into your body and mind.

① Lie on your back.
② Keep your legs hip-width apart. Let your arms lie naturally by the side of your body, palms facing up.
③ Relax your body and take deep, quiet breaths.
④ Let any unnecessary thoughts go. You should feel the tiredness of your body gradually lessening. Two to three minutes should be enough.
⑤ When you feel that you're finished, breathe deeply into your abdomen and hold it, raise your upper body with strength, and go on to the next pose.

This posture is different from just lying down because your mind is focused on the act of lying down. It's a very good way to recover from fatigue, and is most effective when done on a hard surface such as a *tatami* mat or rug.

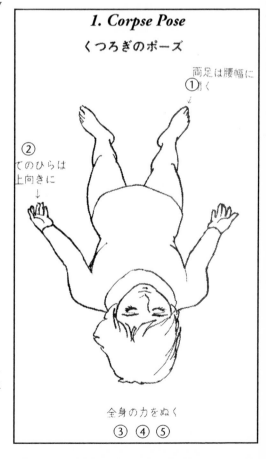

1. Corpse Pose
くつろぎのポーズ

両足は腰幅に
① おく

② てのひらは
上向きに

全身の力をぬく
③ ④ ⑤

2. Cat Pose (Marjaryasana) and 3. Alternative Cat Pose

For anti-aging, stiff and contracted muscles, and to relax the nerves and slim the back, abdomen, hips, and legs.

A stiff back slows down your movements and causes you to age. This posture eliminates muscle stiffness all over the body, especially the back. It was inspired by the movements of cats, the most flexible of all the animals. Cats often yawn and stretch comfortably – this is their "rejuvenation trick." We, too, need to be flexible physically and mentally to maintain youth and beauty. The spine and back muscles are a very important pillar of support for humans, who walk erect.

① Get on your hands and knees.

② Round your back as you breathe out quietly. Pretend you're a cat. Bring your head between your arms.

③ Try to round your back and tighten your abdomen as much as you can as you finish exhaling. Hold your breath for three seconds. When you can't hold any longer, loosen your body as you start inhaling slowly. Come back to the original position on your hands and knees.

④ As you breathe out, begin to arch your back. Go as far as you can and look at the ceiling.

⑤ Slowly come back to the original position as you inhale.

⑥ As an alternative, you can stretch out your hands while doing Cat Pose.

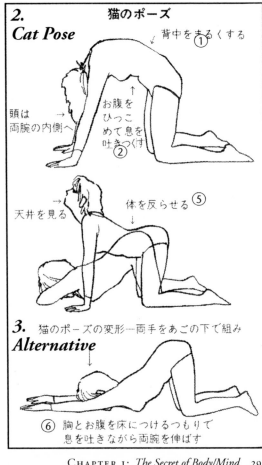

2. Cat Pose 猫のポーズ

背中をまるくする ①

お腹をひっこめて息を吐きつくす ②

頭は両腕の内側へ →

天井を見る → 体を反らせる ⑤

3. Alternative 猫のポーズの変形──両手をあごの下で組み

⑥ 胸とお腹を床につけるつもりで息を吐きながら両腕を伸ばす

3. Forward Bend Pose (Paschimottanasana)

For diabetes, hemorrhoids, impotence, constipation, hypertrophic liver, hypertrophic spleen, fatigue, anti-aging, and slimming the hips and waist.

This posture prevents aging and helps you recover from fatigue, both of which are caused by stiff muscles in the neck and lower back and contracted muscles in the back of the legs. It tones the muscles of the entire abdominal area, helping eliminate fat around the lower abdomen and hips, and also prevents the intestines from expanding, encourages bowel movement, and cures constipation. It cures impotence and frigidity by enhancing blood circulation to the lower body, especially the sex organs, prostate, uterus, rectum, and bladder.

① Sit on the floor with your legs stretched out. Stretch your arms in front and stretch your Achilles tendons as you inhale deeply and focus your attention on your tanden.

② As you exhale, rock your upper body back and forth a few times.

③ Without bending your knees, try to place your abdomen and chest on your thighs, with your head between your knees. Bend forward as far as you can, allowing your hands to go beyond your feet if possible.

④ Grab your big toes and pull to create more stretch in your Achilles tendons. Put your elbows on the floor, and try to bring your upper body toward your feet using your elbows as leverage.

⑤ Keep your focus on your tanden. Exhale as you tighten the muscles around your elbows, and inhale as you relax them. Continue breathing rhythmically in this way. If your legs are very tight, lightly punching the muscles in the back of your legs and feet will help you with the posture.

3. Forward Bend Pose (Paschimottanasana)

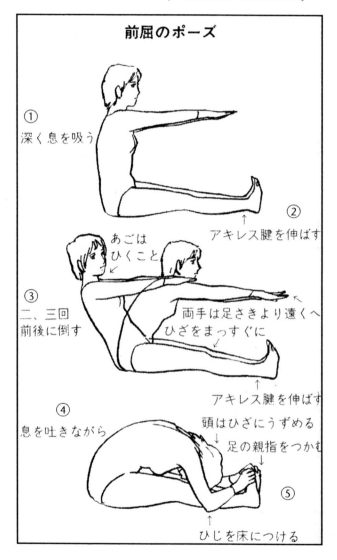

前屈のポーズ

① 深く息を吸う

② アキレス腱を伸ばす

あごは ひくこと

③ 二、三回 前後に倒す

両手は足さきより遠くへ ひざをまっすぐに

アキレス腱を伸ばす

④ 息を吐きながら

頭はひざにうずめる

足の親指をつかむ

⑤

ひじを床につける

4. Cobra Pose (Bhujangasana)

For apathy, lack of self-confidence, pressure in the organs, abnormality of the sex organs, better blood circulation, digestive ability, elimination ability, and beautiful proportion.

Cobra Pose eliminates muscle fatigue in the back, chest, abdomen, and hips, promoting good blood circulation in the spine and sympathetic nerves. It also stimulates the abdominal muscles, making it effective for constipation, and stimulates the sacrum, making it effective for female problems and the promotion of beauty. It also treats nervousness.

① Lie relaxed on your stomach. Bend your arms and place your palms on the floor, centered below your shoulders. The edges of your hands should touch your body.

② Gradually lift your head and upper body as you inhale slowly. Try to use just the strength of your spine, not your arms.

③ Once your upper body is raised, use the strength of your arms to arch back even farther. Don't let your lower abdomen (below the navel) leave the floor.

④ Keep your eyes wide open and stare at a point on the ceiling. Focus your attention on the area of the spine that's feeling pressure.

⑤ Now breathe in as if you're stretching the muscles of the chest, abdomen, and legs even more, and hold your breath for seven to twelve seconds.

⑥ Exhale slowly and relax you body, returning to the original position on the floor.

4. Cobra Pose (Bhujangasana)

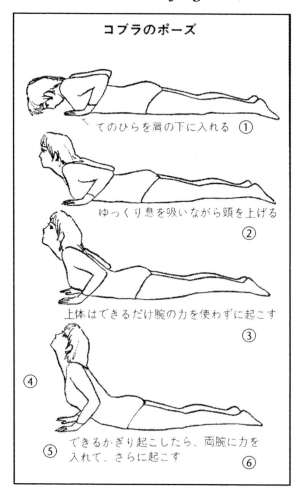

コブラのポーズ

てのひらを肩の下に入れる ①

ゆっくり息を吸いながら頭を上げる ②

上体はできるだけ腕の力を使わずに起こす ③

④

できるかぎり起こしたら、両腕に力を
入れて、さらに起こす ⑤ ⑥

5. *Triangle Pose (Trikonasana)*

For bad posture, dislocation of the internal organs, congestion of the organs, anemia, pain, breathing problems, ringing in the ears, anxiety, and lengthening of the legs.

Triangle Pose treats looseness or stiffness of the muscles in the sides and chest, correcting tilted posture. It enhances the function of the organs that were distorted due to bad posture and enforces the function of the organs of elimination, making it effective for constipation or diarrhea. Constipation and ringing in the ears can be treated just by massaging your side.

If you're unbalanced, tilting either right or left when you stand up straight, it signifies that your nerves are unbalanced, which causes your thinking and emotions to be unnatural and abnormal. This posture gives you the energy to maintain balance of body and mind, and helps you relax.

① Stand with your feet apart, twice as wide as your shoulders. Raise your arms to your shoulders and stretch them out to the side, palms facing down. Keep your arms straight so that they're parallel to the floor.

② Without bending your knees, bend your upper body to the right as you exhale, touching your right ankle with your right fingers. Look up at the tip of your left fingers.

③ Move your left arm parallel to the floor. Breathe deeply. Focus on your spine.

④ Repeat on the left side. Doing both sides counts as one repetition of the exercise.

⑤ You may have difficulty with one side. This means that the muscles on that side are contracted and stiff. Do a couple of extra repetitions on that side. For a beginner, two or three repetitions are sufficient.

5. Triangle Pose (Trikonasana)

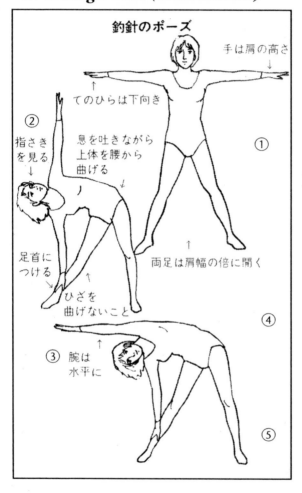

釣針のポーズ

手は肩の高さ

てのひらは下向き

①

② 指さきを見る ↓

息を吐きながら上体を腰から曲げる ↓

足首につける ↓

ひざを曲げないこと ↑

両足は肩幅の倍に開く ↑

④

③ 腕は水平に ↑

⑤

6. Tree Pose (Vrksasana)

For arteriosclerosis, bad posture, fatigue in the internal organs, and slimming and eliminating fat in the legs.

I'd like you to practice this posture in particular if you're not able to balance while standing on one leg. When you stand on one leg, your entire body collaborates to prevent you from falling; therefore, this posture can enhance your ability to maintain balance and harmonize your body and mind.

When you lift your right leg, you stimulate and activate the organs on the left side of your body, such as the stomach, and when you lift your left leg, you stimulate and activate the organs on the right side, such as the liver. This posture can also help you recover from twisting, being off balance, and tilting forward, and it slims your legs. It also enhances your ability to tighten your anus. Because of this, people with only one leg are less likely to suffer from hemorrhoids.

① Stand on your left foot. Place the arch of your right foot against your left thigh, keeping your knee out to the side parallel to the floor. Strengthen your left big toe and the back of your left foot.

② Making sure your back is straight, push your hips slightly forward.

③ Keep your palms together and your elbows parallel to the floor. Take a few deep breaths.

④ As you exhale slowly, bend your left knee and sink down to sit on your leg, with your back straight. Breathe deeply and quietly. Focus your eyes on your fingertips. Repeat several times.

⑤ Repeat on the right leg.

6. Tree Pose (Vrksasana)

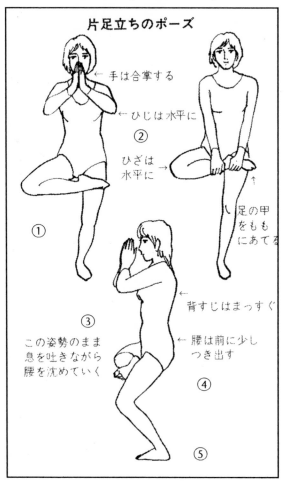

片足立ちのポーズ

← 手は合掌する

← ひじは水平に

②

ひざは
水平に →

①

足の甲
をもも
にあてる

③

背すじはまっすぐ

この姿勢のまま
息を吐きながら
腰を沈めていく

← 腰は前に少し
つき出す

④

⑤

7. Half Lord of the Fishes Pose (Ardha Matsyendrasana)

For neuralgia, inflammation of the organs, bad blood circulation, back pain, pain in the spine, constipation, lack of appetite, and balancing the body by eliminating distortion of the spine.

Your physical and mental activity can be enhanced through spinal twists. Twisting the spine forcefully and then returning it to a normal position treats distortion of the spine, and also enhances blood circulation. When your spine is twisted, you're more likely to have problems such as congestion and inflammation. This posture also stimulates and increases flexibility in the back muscles on both the right and left sides.

① Sit on the floor with your legs in front of you. Bend your left leg and lock it underneath your buttocks.

② Bend your right leg and place your right foot on the outside of the left thigh with the bottom of the foot flat on the floor.

③ Twist your upper body to the right. Place your left elbow on the outside of your right knee and grab your right big toe with your left hand.

④ Keep your right hand on your back. As you exhale, twist your head and upper body to the right as far as possible.

⑤ The angle of your upper body should vary slightly depending on which part of the spine is distorted. If the upper part is distorted, twist your body with your upper body as you tilt forward. If the distortion is in your lower back, twist your upper body as you tilt backward.

⑥ Exhale and tuck in your chin.

⑦ Before your exhale is complete, relax your entire body, letting go of the left hand and coming back to the original position.

⑧ Repeat on the other side. Keep your focus on your spine as you twist two or three times on each side. Try to keep your spine straight.

7. *Half Lord of the Fishes Pose (Ardha Matsyendrasana)*

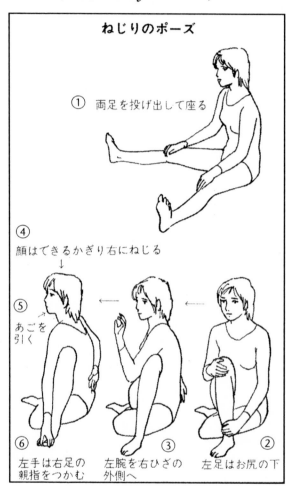

ねじりのポーズ

① 両足を投げ出して座る

④ 顔はできるかぎり右にねじる

⑤ あごを引く

⑥ 左手は右足の親指をつかむ

③ 左腕を右ひざの外側へ

② 左足はお尻の下

8. Traditional Fish Pose (Matsyasana, with legs in Padmasana)

For asthma, bronchitis, cold, constipation, overweight, and beautiful posture. Practice before study or work to activate the nerves in the head.

Fish Pose is effective in eliminating pressure in the chest and stomach area. It also strengthens the lungs by flexing the muscles around the neck and pelvis and stimulates the abdominal muscles and sacrum. It eliminates congestion in the back by sending blood to the neck and spine, and is a good pose for someone who's humpbacked. Because it opens the chest, it makes you feel relaxed and merrier.

① Place the arch of your right foot on top of your left thigh. Then place the arch of your left foot on top of your right thigh, crossing over the right shin. Alternatively, you may place your left leg on the bottom if that's easier for you. This is called *kekka-fuza* (*Padmasana*), or lotus position.

② Slowly lie down in this posture. Exhale and place your elbows on the floor one at a time. Be careful not to fall and hit your head on the floor.

③ Keep your thighs from lifting off the floor.

④ Once the top of your head reaches the floor, let go of your elbows and grab your big toes. Open and lift your chest and arch your back as you breathe in.

⑤ Breathe lightly and focus on your lower abdomen.

8. *Traditional Fish Pose (Matsyasana, with legs in Padmasana)*

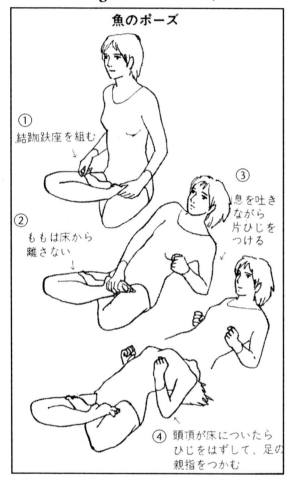

魚のポーズ

① 結跏趺座を組む

② ももは床から離さない

③ 息を吐きながら片ひじをつける

④ 頭頂が床についたらひじをはずして、足の親指をつかむ

9. Plow Pose (Halasana)

For anti-aging, muscle problems, back pain, distortion of the neck, neuralgia, constipation, stomach problems, and promoting beauty by burning fat in the back and stomach.

Plow Pose stretches the muscles of the back completely, promoting flexibility in the back muscles, which helps the spine maintain a normal position. It also strongly contracts and stimulates the abdominal muscles, making it especially good for treating constipation. It also stimulates the sacrum, which improves posture.

This pose is often practiced as part of general exercise and stretching, but in yoga the body is bent more intensely. Practice it every day until you master it.

① Lie on your back. Place your arms by your side with your palms face down. Keep your legs straight together.

② As you slowly exhale, lift your legs to an angle of 45 degrees from the floor, and hold.

③ Lift again until your legs are perpendicular to the floor, and hold. Then lift again until they're parallel to the floor in back of you, and hold. Continue exhaling slowly.

④ Keep your knees straight and your arms on the floor.

⑤ When your feet touch the floor in back of you, stretch your Achilles tendons by moving your heels as far forward as possible. Try to let your chin touch your chest.

⑥ Hold for ten to fifteen seconds, breathing slowly.

⑦ Once you become more flexible, try to bend your knees, bringing them close to your shoulders. This is the perfect position.

9. Plow Pose (Halasana)

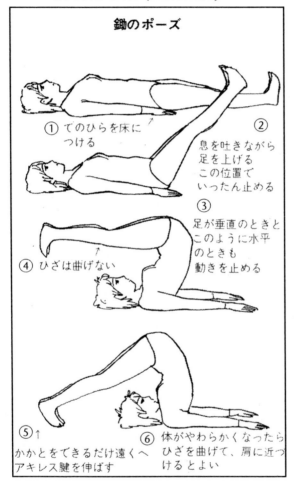

鋤のポーズ

① てのひらを床に つける

② 息を吐きながら 足を上げる この位置で いったん止める

③ 足が垂直のときと このように水平 のときも 動きを止める

④ ひざは曲げない

⑤ ↑ かかとをできるだけ遠くへ アキレス腱を伸ばす

⑥ 体がやわらかくなったら ひざを曲げて、肩に近づ けるとよい

10. Bow Pose (Dhanurasana)

For diabetes, impotence, infertility, irregular menstruation, constipation, rheumatism, overweight, shaping up the bust and hip, and recovery from the fatigue of working in a chair.

Bow Pose activates the endocrine glands and strengthens the entire spine and central nerves. It's also effective for problems in the thyroid glands, thymus, entrance to the liver, and the liver, kidneys, and spleen. It strengthens the gonads, treats frigidity and impotence, and enhances sexual activity. It eliminates unpleasant feelings and makes you more active.

Bow Pose also puts pressure on the abdomen, promotes blood circulation, and strengthens the hips, so it helps you feel refreshed. It's a quick fix for constipation and asthma.

① Lie on your stomach and relax your body.

② Grab your left ankle with both hands and lift your leg two or three times as you exhale. Do the same with the right leg. Do extra repetitions on whichever leg feels more difficult.

③ This time, grab both ankles from the outside. (With practice, you will be able to grab your ankles from the inside.)

④ Point your toes toward the floor and stretch your Achilles tendons, lifting the legs as you breathe out, arching your back, and opening your chest.

⑤ Try to remain in the posture as you breathe slowly and quietly.

⑥ Once you become comfortable with the posture, try rocking your body back and forth like a rocking chair for greater effect.

10. Bow Pose (Dhanurasana)

弓のポーズ

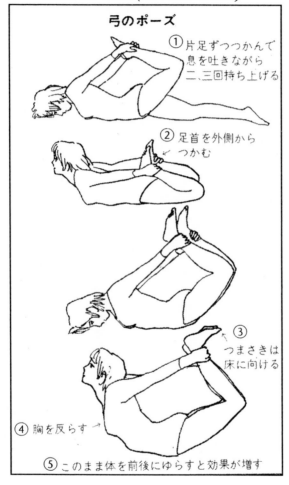

① 片足ずつつかんで
息を吐きながら
二、三回持ち上げる

② 足首を外側から
つかむ

③ つまさきは
床に向ける

④ 胸を反らす

⑤ このまま体を前後にゆらすと効果が増す

11. Grasshopper (Salabhasana)

For *Splanchnoptosis* (prolapsed organs), dislocation of the internal organs, dislocation of the uterus, constipation, irritated mind, lassitude, shaping up and balancing the lower body.

By holding breath and keeping this pose one strengthens lung. Therefore heart, liver, stomach are activated. It also stimulates the abdominal muscle, which solves constipation, irritation, keeps up mental stability, and promotes quickened motions Also this pose fixes humpback posture. As this pose tightens muscles of hip and buttock, tightens waist line, uplift hips, therefore body proportion improves and softens face expression.

① Lie on your stomach with both palm down, making grips softly. Place them under your thighs.

② Place your forehead on the floor and pull your chin in strongly. Lift up your legs one by one. Repeat 2~3 times. This pose must be done with holding the breath with *kimbaku* (holding your breath).

③ Pushing floor with both crunched hands, lift both legs up. Both legs must be stretched all the time. Do not try to lift your legs up high yet but try to lift your pelvis up.

④ Lift up your legs to maximum, hold for more than 10 seconds with your breath also holding. Concentrate your mind on your pelvis and spine. You will be accustomed to it soon even if it is difficult at the beginning.

⑤ Lower down your both legs slowly exhaling gently, then when reaching the floor, release yourself and relax.

11. Grasshopper (Salabhasana)

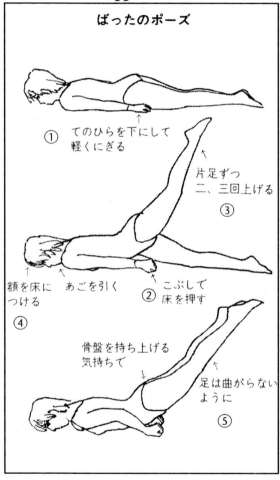

ばったのポーズ

① てのひらを下にして
軽くにぎる

③ 片足ずつ
二、三回上げる

④ 額を床に
つける

あごを引く

② こぶして
床を押す

骨盤を持ち上げる
気持ちで

⑤ 足は曲がらない
ように

12. Upward Bow, or Wheel Pose (Urdhva Dhanurasana)

For impotence, sterility, irregular menstruation, rheumatism, indigestion, constipation, discomfort, and recovery from fatigue.

Wheel Pose activates the endocrine system, especially the sex glands. If the sympathetic nerves are overexcited, it suppresses them, relaxing you and bringing your feelings and desires to a natural state.

For women, it reduces unwanted fat, develops the bust and hips, and slims the waist, making it particularly important for creating a beautiful body.

① Lie on your back. Bend your knees and bring your heels to your buttocks. Place your palms on the floor with your fingers pointing toward your shoulders.

② As you exhale, support your body with the top of your head and your big toes. Slowly stretch your arms and legs to lift your hips.

③ Try to narrow the distance between your hands and feet, and lift your hip as high as you can. Open your chest and lift your chin. Try to look at the floor. Lift your heels and use your toes to shift the weight of your entire body to your head. Straighten your knees.

④ Focus on your pelvis. Continue breathing slowly and quietly as you remain in the pose.

⑤ When you're finished, return to the original position and relax as you take a break. Once you're more advanced, you can enter the posture from an upright position, which is even more effective.

12. Upward Bow, or Wheel Pose (Urdhva Dhanurasana)

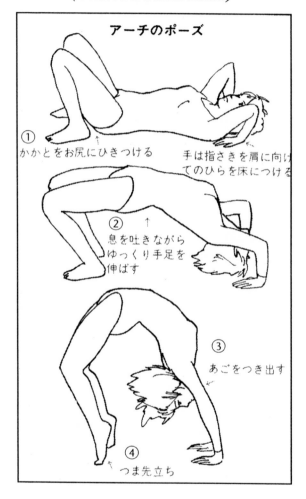

アーチのポーズ

① かかとをお尻にひきつける

手は指さきを肩に向けてのひらを床につける

② 息を吐きながらゆっくり手足を伸ばす

③ あごをつき出す

④ つま先立ち

13. Supported Shoulder Stand Pose
(Salamba Sarvangasana)

For maintaining youth, strengthening sexual ability, enhancing the function of the internal organs, promoting bright skin, correcting the shape of the body, and beautification.

The effect of this posture is just as good as a handstand but it's less difficult, making it great for beginners. It stimulates and strengthens the thyroid gland, which controls stamina, helping prevent decay of the skin and enhancing sexual ability. It sends lots of blood to the spinal nerves so it activates the reflex ability and quickens motions.

① Lie on your back. Place your palms on the floor by your side.

② Slowly lift your legs as you exhale. Keep your knees straight.

③ Lift your lower hips and back, pushing against the floor with your hands. When your hips are high enough, support them with your hands and push up, making your upper body and legs as vertical as possible.

④ Try to keep your chin tucked into your chest. Keep the back of your neck, shoulders, and elbows on the floor to support your body.

⑤ Close your eyes. Focus your attention at your throat, where the thyroid gland is located. Breathe slowly and fully from your tanden.

⑥ Don't try too hard – just hold the posture as long as you can. When you're finished, slowly lower your upper body, then your legs. Don't lower your whole body at once.

⑦ When you're finished, relax, breathing regularly until your pulse returns to normal. Beginners can practice the posture up to three times at first.

13. Supported Shoulderstand Pose (Salamba Sarvangasana)

逆さか立ちのポーズ

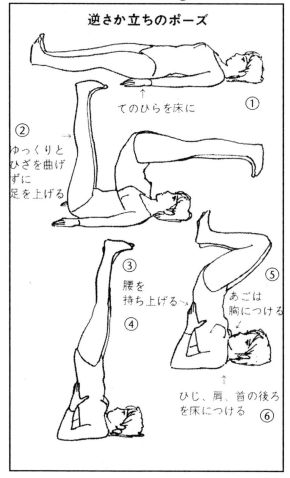

① てのひらを床に

② ゆっくりと
ひざを曲げ
ずに
足を上げる

③ 腰を
持ち上げる

④

⑤ あごは
胸につける

⑥ ひじ、肩、首の後ろ
を床につける

14. Core Power Strengthening Pose

For strengthening the very state of being human, helping to focus your power in your tanden.

Core power is tanden power. Tanden is the center that balances the mind and body. If someone says the martial art term *koshiga haitte inai*, meaning "the center of gravity is not sufficiently low or not in the right place," it means that the energy of the entire body is not concentrated in the tanden. You need to strengthen tanden in order to discipline your mind and body. This is the most important posture of all.

Tanden exists at the center of the triangle that connects lumbar vertebra #3, the rectum, and the navel. Looking from the front, it is located behind the point about four inches below your navel.

① Stand up straight with your legs hip-width apart. Tuck in your chin with your hands behind you, and breathe in with your chest open. Make fists with your thumbs folded in, palm side up.

② Once your chest is full, lift your heels and swing your arms to the front with force, bend your knees slightly, and hold your breath (a practice known as *kumbak*).

③ As you do this, try to focus all your power in your tanden.

④ Hold your breath, maintain the posture, and focus on tanden.

⑤ Straighten your knees and return to the original position.

⑥ In terms of breathing, the key is to inhale slowly and fully into the chest and exhale quickly and forcefully. In other words, align your intention, movement, and focus.

14. Core Power Strengthening Pose

中心力強化のポーズ

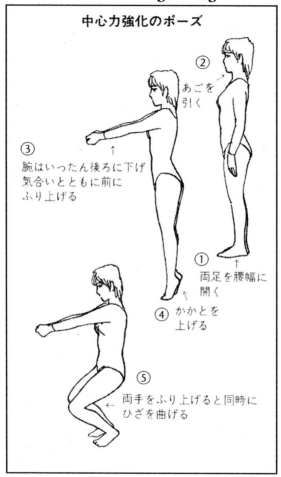

② あごを引く

③ 腕はいったん後ろに下げ気合いとともに前にふり上げる

① 両足を腰幅に開く

④ かかとを上げる

⑤ 両手をふり上げると同時にひざを曲げる

15. Peacock Pose (Mayurasana)

For eliminating congestion in the internal organs such as the stomach and liver, strengthening the internal organs, countering aging of the body and mind, and maintaining a youthful body and an upbeat attitude.

In Peacock Pose, your elbows put pressure on your chest and stomach, stimulating the organs and treating poor blood circulation. The pose also activates the abdominal arteries, counteracting their calcification – one of the biggest causes of aging and high blood pressure – and strengthens the autonomic nerves by stimulating the neck and the entire spine.

Peacock Pose stabilizes the emotions naturally, opening the door to a more positive life. It straightens the spine and makes your face brighter, allowing your unique and charming personality to manifest in your heart and your appearance.

① Get down on all fours with your knees spread and your fingers pointing toward your feet.

② Keep your knees shoulder-width apart, elbows touching the lower abdomen. Slowly shift your weight onto your elbows.

③ Lower your head and touch the floor with your forehead. Support your upper body with your forehead and hands and straighten your legs, with your hands acting as a stem. Straighten your feet as well, not just your knees.

④ Lift your forehead and push your chin forward. As you breathe in, push your body forward, shifting your weight to the front.

⑤ When your legs have lifted from the floor naturally, support your body with your elbows, lift your legs as if you're balancing, and hold your breath (a practice known as *kumbak*). Keep your back straight and hold the posture with your body floating parallel to the floor.

⑥ Hold the posture as long as possible. When you've finished, relax for a while.

15. Peacock Pose (Mayurasana)

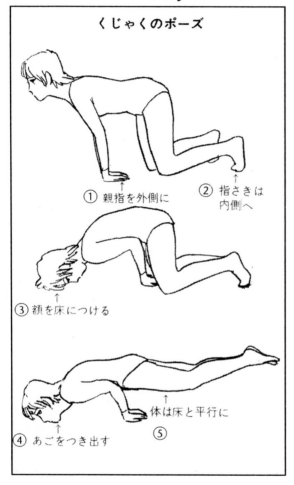

くじゃくのポーズ

① 親指を外側に

② 指さきは
内側へ

③ 額を床につける

④ あごをつき出す

⑤ 体は床と平行に

16. Supported Headstand Pose (Salamba Sirsasana)

For headache, insomnia, indigestion, problems in the sex organs, asthma, nervousness, stiff shoulder, stomachache, back pain, and problems of the eye, ear, and nose. Also helps students enhance their memory.

Problems caused by our upright position can be treated by reversing the body. Because we walk on our feet and are subject to gravity, our blood doesn't circulate to the brain sufficiently. Headstand Pose strengthens your neck – a critical connection between your brain and your internal organs. When the function of vagus nerves in the neck is enhanced, the internal organs become more active as well, and more blood flows to the brain, helping you recover from fatigue more quickly.

①Kneel down and interlace your fingers on the floor. Place your head inside your hands and slowly lift your hips, focusing on balancing your legs.

②Try to bring your feet closer to your head as you shift your weight to your head.

③With your back straight, lift your feet slightly off the floor. Lift your legs gracefully, bend your knees, and hold. Avoid kicking the floor as you would in an athletic sport.

④Slowly straighten your legs as you exhale slowly. Ideally, your entire body would be vertical. Find your center by moving your legs slightly.

⑤Keep breathing deeply and quietly. If your mind wanders, your body will collapse, so keep your focus. Hold the posture as long as possible – five seconds is long enough for beginners. Even if you can't manage this, your effort counts.

16. Supported Headstand Pose
(Salamba Sirsasana)

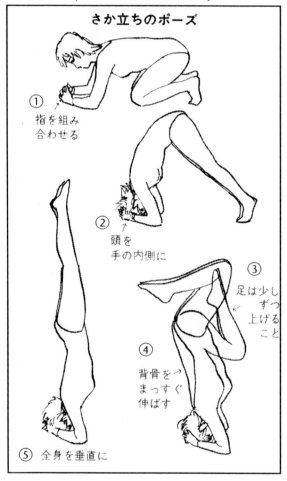

さか立ちのポーズ

① 指を組み
合わせる

② 頭を
手の内側に

③ 足は少し
ずつ
上げる
こと

④ 背骨を→
まっすぐ
伸ばす

⑤ 全身を垂直に

III. PEACE OF MIND WITH ZAHO

Zaho stabilizes your mind and enhances concentration

Zaho is usually practiced during meditation. It helps stabilize the mind, enhances concentration, and corrects physical problems.

What's really important in meditation is correct posture. When your posture is balanced, your breath is steadier and peace of mind increases.

When the body is distorted, the cerebrum senses an abnormal stimulation. It becomes fatigued as a result, and unable to function naturally.

When your posture is correct, your upper body is relaxed and your energy is naturally drawn to the legs, hips, and lower abdomen. In other words, your energy is focused primarily in your tanden, and when energy is in your tanden, your cerebrum is balanced and your nerves active.

What I'd like you to learn in zaho is the right condition of mind – you're your mind is natural and flowing smoothly, not blocked or stuck. To achieve this, begin by practicing how to focus, going into a state of nothingness and then letting your mind be natural.

I will discuss meditation later, but first I'd like to mention *seishin-toitsu* (mental concentration, or unification of the mind and spirit). You begin mental concentration by focusing on an object, such as the tip of a candle flame, the smell of incense, the sound of a watch ticking, and so on. Then shut out everything else completely. If you focus on the sound of a watch, for example, try to listen to just the ticking, without hearing the breeze from outside or the noise of cars.

Our brain cannot think or feel two things at once. Determine an object to focus your mind on.

As you advance in this training, you will realize that your consciousness and senses have become sharper, while at the same time your mind is calmer and more relaxed. How is such a contradictory phenomenon possible?

This is a natural state of the human body and mind, but you can't experience it when you're leading a lazy life. It's the same with the Buddhist teaching that you can't attain power without a completely relaxed state of mind.

Three warnings about practicing Zaho

When you practice focusing, you shouldn't strain yourself as you do when you want to work or study efficiently. When your body and mind are stiff, your brain resists, which distracts your focus.

There are various controlling points in our brain that react to different stimulations so that it will work while distracted.

If you focus your attention or consciousness on one thing without straining, you can bring these separate controlling points together in collaboration with each other.

In this way, the entire brain can react to one excited state simultaneously, creating the ultimate excited state, accompanied by the ultimate stillness.

You practice zaho in order to get to this state quickly – but there are some rules you must follow (in addition to not straining, as mentioned previously).

1. Lengthen your neck, as if you're being pulled up by your hair and you're trying to penetrate the sky with your head.
2. Open your chest to the right and left sides and lift it up.
3. Stretch your stomach top and bottom, pulling it slightly. Make *rectus abdominis* in your abdomen like a stick straight from bottom to top. Push your pelvis up.

If you follow these three rules, you will effectively store force in your tanden.

As a result, your sphincter will tighten naturally, your spine will be straight, your chest open, and your brain relaxed – a perfect condition for concentrating your mind. Store force only in your tanden, relaxing all your other muscles.

Here are some self-check methods you can use to determine if you're doing zaho correctly.

1. Your breath is naturally deep, quiet, and strong.
2. Your upper body is relaxed and your mind is relaxed and calm.
3. Your lower body is filled with force, making your body feel full and stable.
4. You senses are acute, you're aware of all directions, your consciousness is clear, and your mind is stable.

When you practice *dozenko*, or moving zen practice, in this condition, your yoga practice will be most effective.

People often complain that their legs fall asleep, they have back pain, or their shoulders are tense when they practice zaho. When you find yourself in this situation, pull up your head and straighten your back. These symptoms happen because your spine is in an unstable position.

1. Seiza-ho

For flexibility of the joints and muscles of the legs and stability of mind. (*Seiza* means "correct" sitting in Japanese. To sit *seiza-style*, kneel on the floor and fold your legs underneath your thighs while resting your buttocks on your heels (as in Lion Pose, or *Simhasana*).

① Sit in seiza. Cross the first toes and keep your knees together.
② Pull your hips all the way back as you breathe in. Keep your spine straight.
③ Place your palms firmly on the base of your thighs, and lift your knees.
④ With force in tanden, drop your knees to the floor and let them open naturally, in correspondence to the openness of your pelvis. Knowing the correct angle of your legs is the basis for a stable seiza practice.
⑤ Place your palms on your thighs. Relax your upper body. Breathe deeply and quietly.

2. Kekka-fuza, or Lotus Pose (Padmasana)

For flexibility of the joints and muscles of the legs, strengthening concentration, balancing the internal organs.

① Sit with your legs in front of you, knees straight. Bend whichever leg is easier and place that foot on the base of the opposite thigh with the sole of the foot facing up. Try to pull the heel closer to your lower abdomen.
② Place the foot of the other leg on top of the opposite thigh to cross your legs. Try not to let the knees lift up. If you feel like you're falling backward, you can place a cushion under your buttocks.
③ Create circles with your thumbs and index fingers, keeping the other fingers straight. This is called *mudra*. Place your hands on your knees with your palms facing up. Relax your upper body and focus on your tanden.

1. Seiza-ho
2. Kekka-fuza, or Lotus Pose (Padmasana)

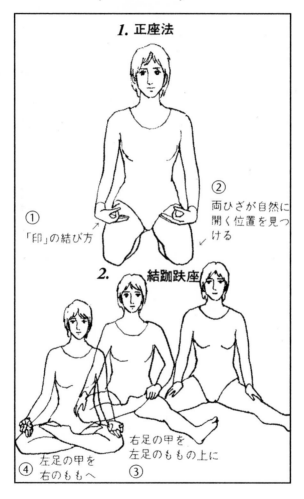

1. 正座法

② 両ひざが自然に
開く位置を見つ
ける

① 「印」の結び方

2. 結跏趺座

右足の甲を
左足のももの上に

④ 左足の甲を
右のももへ

③

3. Hanka-fuza, or Half Lotus Pose (Ardha Padmasana, or Ardha Kamalasana)

For flexibility of the back muscles and to maintain balance of the hormones and nerves.

① From a seated position, bend the leg that's more difficult to bend, and place the foot at the base of the opposite leg.

② Place this leg on top of the bent leg and pull it close to your lower abdomen.

③ Form a mudra with both hands as you did in *Kekka-fuza,* or Lotus Pose (*Padmasana*) and place your hands on your knees. Keep your spine straight and relax your neck, shoulders, back, elbows, and wrists. Let your armpits open slightly. Focus on your tanden and breathe deeply and slowly.

4. Stable Sitting Pose (Siddhasana for men and Siddha Yoni Asana for women)

For correcting problems in the pelvis and for flexibility of the muscles in the lower body.

① From a seated position, bend the knee that's more difficult to bend and place your heel at the perineal area (between the sex organs and anus).

② Bend the opposite leg and try to pull the heel toward the arch of the other foot.

③ Try to align the three spots – perineum and two heels – on a line.

5. Yogic Sitting Pose (Swastikasana)

For strengthening the knee joints and muscles of the legs and for stability of mind.

① From a seated position, bend the leg that's easier to bend, and pull the heel in toward the perineum.

② Bend the opposite leg and place the heel on top of the other heel.

③ Straighten your back muscles and focus your mind on your tanden as you breathe deeply and quietly.

3. Hanka-fuza, or Half Lotus Pose (Ardha Padmasana, or Ardha Kamalasana)

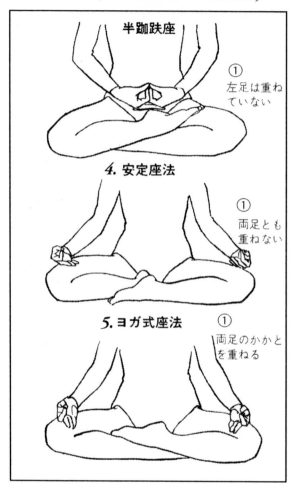

半跏趺座

① 左足は重ね
ていない

4. 安定座法

① 両足とも
重ねない

5. ヨガ式座法

① 両足のかかと
を重ねる

6. Bound Angle Pose (Baddha Konasana)

For flexibility of the muscles of the legs and to correct problems in the pelvis.

① Sit with your legs stretched wide apart. Bend your knees and bring the bottoms of your feet together.

② Grab your toes with your hands and pull your heels toward your body, keeping your back straight.

③ Try to keep your knees on the floor as much as possible.

7. Resting Seated Pose

For correcting the balance of hormones and nerves and for stability of mind.

① From a seated position, bend the leg that's more difficult to bend, and place that heel at the bottom of the opposite thigh, close to the buttocks. Bend the other leg and stand with your knee aligned with your nose.

② Interlace your hands around the knee that's lifted, pulling it toward your chest.

8. Knee Standing Pose

For brain activity and to strengthen concentration.

① Kneel, with your knees slightly more than shoulder-width apart. The tips of your feet should be slightly wider than your knees.

② Make a fist with your right hand with the thumb folded in and wrap your fist in your left hand. Hold it slightly above the solar plexus.

③ Keep your elbows out, arms horizontal. Keep your body straight.

④ Meditate, lightly touching your chin with your fist, eyes half open.

6. Bound Angle Pose (Baddha Konasana)

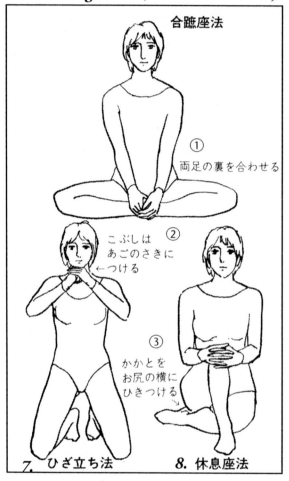

合蹠座法

① 両足の裏を合わせる

② こぶしは
あごのさきに
←つける

③ かかとを
お尻の横に
ひきつける

7. ひざ立ち法

8. 休息座法

9. Chair Sitting Pose

For strengthening the function of the hormones and nerves.

① Choose a chair that's comfortable for you. Sit with your knees at 90 degrees, lower legs perpendicular to the floor.

② Keep your feet and knees together and place your hands on your thighs.

③ Bring your hands to your hips and lift your knees as you inhale. Hold your breath and focus your energy in the lower abdomen. Your knees will naturally open to maintain balance. Bring your knees down in this position.

④ Energize your big toes and the inner side of the knees, and make *Jnana Mudra* (touch your index fingers and thumbs) with your hands on your thighs.

10. Hero Pose (Virasana)

For hip joints, knee joints, ankles, and flexibility of the muscles of the legs.

① Sit in seiza.

② Bring your lower legs to the outside of the thighs.

③ Sit between your thighs, with your toes pointing out.

④ Keep your knees on the floor.

⑤ Rest your hands lightly on your thighs.

9. Chair Sitting Pose
10. Hero Pose (Virasana)

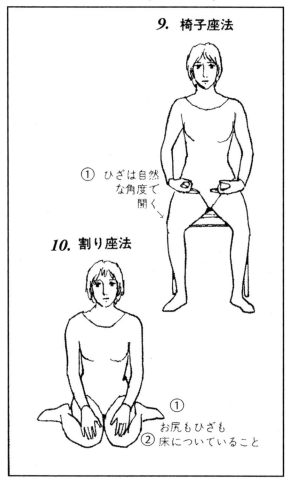

9. 椅子座法

① ひざは自然な角度で開く

10. 割り座法

①
② お尻もひざも床についていること

11. Kongo-Gassho, or Salutation Seal (Anjali Mudra or Hrdayanjali Mudra)

For energizing, strengthening of the vagus and sympathetic nerves, balancing, and enhancing the function of the autonomic nerves.

This is a good *gassho* (salutation seal) for any type of zaho.

① Separate the thumbs, keeping the fingers together to form a gassho. Keep a small amount of space between the lower palms.

② Breathe forcefully, as if breathing with tanden, filling your knees with force.

③ Strengthen just the middle fingers in gassho, relaxing the others. The middle fingers are directly connected to the spine. Raise the hands in gassho so that the tips of the middle fingers are in front of the tip of your nose.

④ Keep your elbows slightly below shoulder level.

12. Gassho Sadhana (Ascetic Training) (palms together with the Prayer's Heart)

For enhancing the ability to internalize consciousness.

① Form a *gassho* by creating a triangle with your thumbs and the other fingers. Tighten your sphincter and inhale deeply.

② Relax your thumbs, keeping the center of the triangle at eye level, and look through the triangle at an object, such as a candle flame.

③ Let your conscious mind imagine the form of God, or something else of your choosing.

This is usually practiced during meditation. Do this with *Kekka-fuza*, or Lotus Pose (*Padmasana*) or *Hanka-fuza*, or Half Lotus Pose (*Ardha Padmasana* or *Ardha Kamalasana*)

11. Kongo-Gassho, or Salutation Seal (Anjali Mudra or Hrdayanjali Mudra)

12. Gassho Sadhana (Ascetic Training) (palms together with the Prayer's Heart)

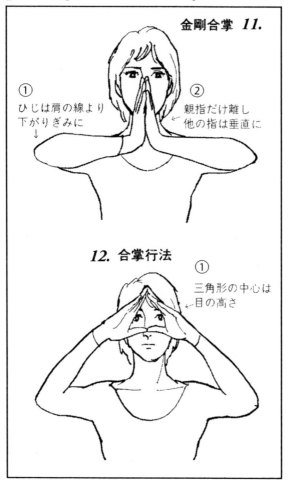

金剛合掌 *11.*

① ひじは肩の線より 下がりぎみに
↓

② 親指だけ離し 他の指は垂直に

12. 合掌行法

① 三角形の中心は 目の高さ

Chapter 2

Nutrients of the Mind and Body

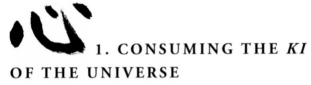

1. CONSUMING THE *KI* OF THE UNIVERSE

Nutrients are taken in through the nose, mouth, and head

Asanas are about postures – in other words, how you use your body. In this chapter, I'll explain the third step of yoga: *pranayama. Ki* is energy. You already know that we take in nutrients through the mouth and nose, but in this case those nutrients are slightly different than the food and oxygen we normally think of. Nutrients that enter through our head – in other words, knowledge – are one part.

This method cultivates the fundamental power you need to practice and balance the postures of the mind and body that were discussed previously. In my understanding, *pranayama* is to nurture ourselves from within. *Prana* is a Hindi word that means *ki* – the active energy of the universe, which travels in and out of our body through our mouth, nose, skin, and head.

This energy exists all over the universe, sustaining all animals and plants on the earth. When we eat food, breathe air, or gain knowledge, we take the active force of the universe into our body. Food is the ki of the earth, air is the ki of the sky, and knowledge is holy ki.

In order to absorb the necessary vital force, we take in air through our nose, mouth, and skin; food through our mouth; and knowledge through our head. We take the most nutritious matter that exists through our mouth, nose, and head, and utilize it.

Pranayama describes in detail how to use certain techniques to achieve specific results.

Breath changes our body and mind

In general, the quality of the air you breathe differs in different places. Have you ever traveled to a Buddhist temple in the mountains where monks train, such as Koyasan in Kyoto, Japan? If so, you must have noticed that the air and atmosphere there is different from what you normally experience in the city or at your office.

The air must certainly have made you tense up. That's because the energy of monks training there for hundreds of years still remains. Samurai warriors are said to have felt Sakki, or the hint of kill in the air. The tension may also be caused by differences in the atmosphere. *Yamabushi* (mountain monks) sit under a waterfall when they train, but their training really begins when they experience the atmosphere of the mountain they climb.

I'm sure you can see how breathing that sort of air influences our body and mind compared to the air on a crowded street or the stagnant air in an office.

According to a logical, scientific Western viewpoint, an individual is independent of the world, and has the will to decide whether or not they're influenced by outside forces. But this is wrong.

When we stand in the midst of other people, tables and chairs, flowers and food, everything in the environment influences our body and mind constantly. The air in a particular spot has an enormous influence on our body and mind. If you breathe solemn air, such as at a funeral, your body and mind become tense.

Everyone breathes differently, with a different method.

When you're happy, you breathe like you're happy, but when you're sad, you breathe like you're sad. It's the same with animals. Breath is the language of life. Therefore, if you change your breath, your mood changes as well.

For example:

A. Exhale forcefully when you want to relax.
B. Breathe slowly and quietly when you want to calm your mind.
C. When your chest muscles are tight, causing an imbalance of the adrenal cortex hormone, you feel unpleasant. Arch your upper body back with force, and breathe deeply.
D. When your kidneys are weak, you feel anxious. Stretch back while you breathe.
E. When you're feeling undetermined, bring strength into your legs and abdomen and breathe quickly and forcefully.

Breath can be a key to controlling our body and mind. Our breath changes before our body and mind change – so if you correct your breath, you can be healthy. To heal chronic diseases, begin by changing your breath. If you occasionally become slightly sick, it's generally due to shallow and incomplete breathing.

Deep breathing is the most important thing. Make a point of breathing deeply whenever you can. And breathe completely – not just into your chest (thoracic breathing), but into your abdomen as well (abdominal breathing). Relax your shoulders, neck, and hands during abdominal breathing. This is how to truly relax.

Well-known abdominal breathing techniques include *Kiai* (a vocalization of the fighting spirit that involves special breathing) and laughing breath.

Breath is the key to everything

Let's look at breath in more detail.

When we're surprised, we don't breathe. We breathe in, and then the surprise hits us. Our breath doesn't slow down because we calm down; rather, we calm down naturally once our breath slows down.

Think of laughing and you'll understand this point. We can't laugh on an inhalation. When you laugh, you're exhaling. Conversely, when you're surprised or crying, you're inhaling. In other words, you can sometimes surprise yourself with your own inhalation.

This is even true for animals. When a cat hisses in a fight, it exhales the air that it inhaled deeply, waiting for the moment to attack.

For a long time, understanding the breath has been key to the spirit of various martial and performing arts. Breath is very important in everything. A so-called ma, or an interval of breath that is solid.

Recently, I taught professors at Toho University how to play the violin, even though I myself had never played violin or piano.

You may be wondering what and how I taught them. I simply corrected their irregular breathing. I told them to lift their elbow, or to bend their right elbow. This changed their movement, posture, and brain function, ultimately changing their breath.

This is an application of pranayama. Since I couldn't correct their breathing one by one, I simply instructed them to utilize postures and movements that would automatically correct their breath. They all remarked that within a half hour their performance had improved a great deal.

Diet changes our body and mind

The way you eat determines how you live your life. If you overeat, you become fat, have stomach problem, and become drowsy. Too many cold drinks hurt your stomach and cause indigestion. A moderate amount of alcohol might be good for your body, but an excessive amount damages your internal organs.

There's a very wide and deep connection between the condition of your body and mind and how you eat and drink. Just as different ways of breathing can change your body and mind, so can different ways of eating. Some foods make you fat without your knowing, and some make you aggressive. Your life can be better or worse depending on how and what you eat.

However, let me emphasize that I'm not preaching the art of gourmet eating. Of course, it feels better to eat something that tastes good, but I want to remind you that we don't live just to eat.

If you consume an appropriate amount of food that contains the appropriate nutrients for you, you won't get sick.

Whatever doesn't suit you or is unnecessary becomes toxic. Even something that's good for you can be unhealthy if you eat too much or too little of it.

Food is medicine. If you eat a balanced diet, you're certain to be healthy. If you're sick, eat what your symptoms tell you to eat, and don't eat anything unnecessary. This is the way to make your diet a healing diet.

Taking in nutrients through your head

Choki-ho (harmonizing ki, or the way to control prana through breathing) also teaches you to be aware of the nutrition that you absorb through your head. This may sound strange to you, but let me explain.

When we think, we use only the information that's already in our head. If that includes incorrect knowledge and understanding, we can get confused and make inappropriate decisions.

For example, suppose you have a cold and a fever, and all you know are certain ideas such as it's not good to have a fever, you should take an antipyretic, or you should cool down your head. But there are different types of fever: fevers that need to be left alone and fevers that need to be cooled down. If your knowledge is incorrect, you could end up making your condition worse.

You take in nutrients through your head by studying, reading, and listening to other people in order to acquire the correct understanding about yourself and humans as a whole. But you need to figure out for yourself what to study and what to read, because just as everyone's body constitution and condition differs, we all have our unique ways of studying and different preferences in books.

One thing I will say is that, just like breathing and eating, you need to have a proper "routine" for reading. Reading for a few hours a day is necessary, like meals. These are the three essential nutrients for our body and mind.

2. LAUGHING IS THE BASIS OF BREATHING

The best way to breath is to sing

I have fasted for sixty days with nothing but water. We can live for a while without eating, but what would happen if we stopped breathing? We couldn't survive for five minutes.

We begin breathing as soon as we're born and stop breathing when we die. That's why we say that breath is the source of life. Breath has held this place of importance for a long time. In Japanese, iki-ru, to live, is derived from iki-suru, to breathe. And because long deep breathing is good for our health, nagaiki-suru, longevity, is derived from nagaiki, long breath.

But we may not always take long deep breaths unless we're trained to do so. Many factors in this society make us tense and aggressive. When our body is tilted forward, our breath becomes shallow. We need exercise to relax our mind as well as to correct our posture. When our posture is good, we can take deep, perfect breaths that make us healthy, with a balanced pulse and blood pressure.

In this section, I introduce ten exercises that teach you to breathe deeply with good posture. If you keep practicing and allow this kind of breathing to become a habit, you will dramatically improve your ability to maintain your health.

Yogic breathing always includes both thoracic and abdominal breathing. This is an ideal way of breathing that enables you to take in much more oxygen than the thoracic breathing that's usually practiced in Western exercise.

In abdominal breathing you breathe deeply, all the way down to the bottom of your abdomen. Laughter, yawning, and *Kiai* (a vocalization of the fighting spirit that involves special breathing) are activities that typically make use of abdominal breathing. So is singing.

These are ideal ways to breathe because they're long and deep. Since ancient times, we have used the saying "Laughter is the best medicine," and the act of reciting Chinese poems to a tune with special breathing or practicing *Utai,* a very specialized traditional Japanese way of singing, have long been considered good for longevity because we naturally breathe well while we relax and enjoy.

Yawning is part of our natural ability to maintain balance of body and mind. It's an automatic reflex that supplies the brain with oxygen whenever there's a shortage.

Kiai can also be made much stronger by practicing breathing.

What's important in abdominal breathing is to focus on your tanden and relax your upper body, especially your neck, shoulders, and elbows – to be completely relaxed.

One trick while doing breathing exercises is to relax your entire body and pretend you've become a balloon. Inhale as you loosen your entire body, and exhale by squeezing out the air.

When you inhale, expand your chest as much as possible and when you exhale, contract your abdomen. But don't exert yourself or you can create problems such as headaches due to dilated submucosal vessels.

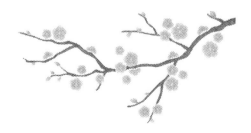

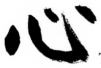 **TEN BREATHING TECHNIQUES**

1. Breathing Exercise A

Stretches the respiratory muscles and strengthens the ability of ribs to expand and contract. Allows you to breathe deeply and naturally, and enhances metabolism.

① With your feet shoulder-width apart, lift and stretch your arms to the side at shoulder level, palms facing the floor. Inhale deeply and quietly through your nose.

② As you exhale slowly through your mouth, bend your right elbow and place your right hand under your armpit, keeping your left arm straight with the palm facing down, and bend your upper body to the left. Turn your neck to look at your left toes.

③ Bring your upper body back to center and inhale slowly and deeply. Repeat on the right side.

2. Breathing Exercise B

① With your feet hip-width apart, lift and stretch your arms in front of your body. Inhale slowly and deeply through your nose.

② Twist your upper body to the right as you exhale. Inhale and twist to the left.

3. Breathing Exercise C

① Stand with your legs hip-width apart. Bend forward as far as you can and, with your arms stretched out, twist your wrists to the inside as you exhale.

② As you inhale, straighten your body and step forward with your right foot, arching your back and lifting your arms.

③ Bring your right foot back to the original position and repeat step 2 with your left foot.

1. Breathing Exercise A

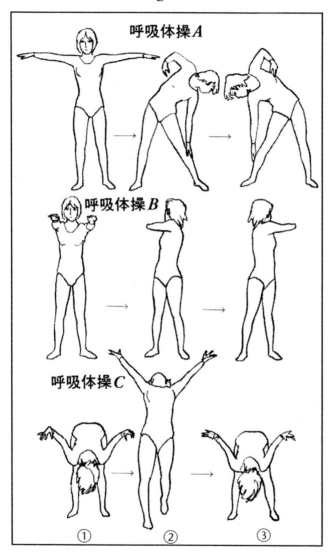

呼吸体操A

呼吸体操B

呼吸体操C

① ② ③

4. Perfect Breathing Technique

The basic *pranayama* technique to control your breath. The fundamental breathing technique.

① Stand with your feet hip-width apart or sit in seiza.

② Inhale through your nose, breathing into the bottom of the lungs as if pushing down the diaphragm. Your abdomen will expand to the front. Next, open your chest wide and breathe into the middle part of the lungs. Breathe in some more, filling up your lungs with air. Next, lift your shoulders and breathe into the collarbone area. Your lower abdomen will sink a little. Do this series of movements continuously, trying to expand the entire chest area gently from the bottom up, diaphragm to collarbone.

③ Practice kumbak (hold the breath) for a few seconds, using the following method: Exhaling slightly, push the air down into your lower abdomen. Next, relax your shoulders and solar plexus, keeping your hips and lower abdomen strong, while you hold the rest of the air. Touch your tongue to the roof of the mouth and focus your mind.

④ Contract your lower abdomen as you exhale, squeezing the air from your body with force in your feet and abdominal muscles. You'll find yourself tilting forward slightly.

⑤ Once you've exhaled 80% of the air, relax your abdomen and feet slightly and straighten your back, allowing inhalation to occur naturally.

5. Kumbak (holding the breath)

Strengthens nerves and latent abilities. After completing perfect breathing (above), inhale, repeat *kumbak*, and do the following:

① Lung muscles stimulation method: Bend back slightly and pound your chest with your fists as you slowly exhale.

② Rib stretching method: Pull your elbows back and expand your chest. Repeat.

③ Ribcage expanding method: Push your hands out in front of you with your arms straight. Keeping them at shoulder height, bring them to your sides. Repeat several times.

④ Forward and back bend method: Bend your upper body forward and back repeatedly.

⑤ *Prana method:* Hold your breath and rotate your arms in a big motion. Close your eyes and continue to hold your breath forcefully until your abdominal area trembles and you begin to perspire – but don't overstrain.

6. Purifying Breathing Technique

For recovering from tiredness. Allows clear air into the lungs, cleanses the blood, stimulates the nerves and hormonal glands, and activates the organs. Try this after any breathing practice.

③ After completing perfect breathing, hold your breath for a few seconds.

③ Pucker your lips as if whistling and exhale little by little. Don't let your cheeks expand. When you've exhaled about half the air, hold your breath again.

③ Exhale the rest of the air in the same manner, but more forcefully. Pretend you're exhaling all the old matter in your body.

7. *Sukha Purbhak, or Nadi Shodhana Pranayama*

Tones the body. Begin by practicing ten times, once in the morning and once at night, then increase the number of repetitions.

① Sit in Seiza position, if possible, with your spine straight and eyes closed.

② Close your left nostril with your left thumb and gently breathe in through your right nostril.

③ Keeping the left nostril shut, close your right nostril with the left ring finger and hold your breath for about 10 seconds (not to the point of discomfort).

④ Lift your left thumb and slowly exhale through your left nostril.

⑤ Once you've exhaled completely, gently breathe in through your left nostril. Close your left nostril with your thumb and hold your breath.

⑥ Lift your ring finger and slowly exhale through your right nostril.

The ideal ratio of breathing in this exercise is inhale for 1, hold for 4, and exhale for 2. In other words, you could also inhale for 2, hold for 8, and exhale for 4. Once you're more comfortable with the exercise, you can inhale for 4, hold for 16, and exhale for 8.

As you do practice this exercise, slowly chant the sacred mantra *"OM"* in your mind. Breathe in as if you're breathing in the mind of God, and breathe out as if you're exhaling filth from your body.

If you practice this breathing technique regularly, your body will become toned, your face will look brighter, and your voice will even sound better.

7. *Sukha Purbhak,* or *Nadi Shodhana Pranayama*

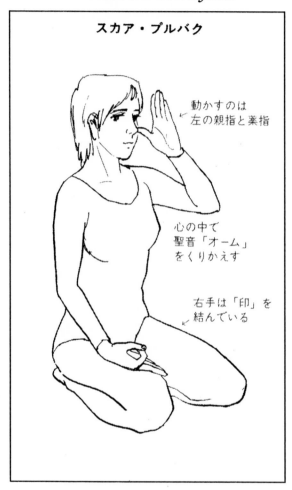

スカア・プルバク

動かすのは
左の親指と薬指

心の中で
聖音「オーム」
をくりかえす

右手は「印」を
結んでいる

8. *Bhramari*

Enables you to listen to the spiritual voice within you. Practice this in a quiet place.

① Sit in Seiza position, if possible, with your spine straight.

② Inhale and exhale rapidly through your nose, making a vibrating sound like a bee.

Alternative method

① Close your ears with your thumbs and breathe in through your nose.

② Hold your breath as long as possible, then exhale.

9. *Kabalabati*

Prevents aging, clears the nerves and glands, cures problems caused by cold.

Sit in *Kekka-fuza* (Lotus Pose, or Padmasana), *Hanka-fuza* (Half Lotus Pose, or *Ardha Padmasana* or *Ardha Kamalasana*), or any yoga meditation position. Keep your back and neck straight.

① Inhale through your nose and stick out your stomach. Immediately relax your abdominal muscles and slowly exhale through your nose as you tighten your stomach.

② Repeat. Try to breathe out more attentively (with mindfulness) than you breathe in.

10. Body and Mind Stabilizing Breathing Technique

Balances the degree of stiffness or looseness of the muscles on the left and right sides of the back, makes the muscles flexible, eliminates distortion of the body and mind.

①Stand with your feet about one foot apart, back straight.

②Inhale through your nose using perfect breathing technique, and hold.

③Place your hands on your waist and twist your upper body left and right while holding your breath. Do this movement quietly and rhythmically three times on each side.

④Still holding the breath, bend your upper body forward and back.

⑤Twist your body left and right one more time.

⑥With your hands still on your waist, slowly exhale.

This technique helps relax your body and mind following a period of focus. Swinging your body back and forth and side to side with your breath held is called *Yodoho* ("swaying method" in Japanese).

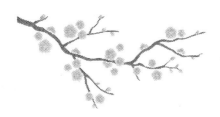

A method to help others heal through breathing

Once you've completely mastered these breathing techniques, you can heal not just your own problems, but those of others as well by giving them your ki or prana.

Place your hands on the troubled parts of the patient's body and imagine that ki is flowing from your hands to them, and pray that they're going to get better. Hold you breath. (Think how mothers often say, "Pain, pain, go away!" when their children are injured – it can be unexpectedly effective!)

You can also direct your ki to a part of your body that's in need. For example, if your heart is weak, sit in seiza and close your eyes. Place your hand on your heart area and breathe deeply and quietly. Then hold your breath and imagine that ki is flowing to your heart. Distinctly visualize your heart as lively and active. As you exhale, affirm that the afflicted parts are cured.

Recently, a young man had a blood transfusion for a friend, and the needle left a big mark and swelling on his arm. The doctor said it would last about a week. I taught him this technique, and the swelling was gone in about an hour. If you haven't experienced this for yourself, you might think it's just a trick, but it's actually effective.

In Japanese, we use the word teate, meaning to treat (literally, to put a hand over the diseased part, and the word teokura, meaning too late (literally, hand lateness or tardiness). But placing your own hands on something is actually the basic of *teate* (hands-on healing).

3. ELIMINATE DISTRESS THROUGH DIET

When we eat, we consume the energy of the universe

We often think incorrectly that food is equal to nutrition, but food alone doesn't produce the force we need to live and sustain our lives. After all, by this same token, food can't provide nutrients to the dead.

If you eat something your body doesn't need naturally, it won't become nutrition for you. If you eat something that you think tastes bad, it will become toxic to your body.

Nutritional power is created only when food and our life force, which gains nutrition from food, are in a cooperative relationship. Food can be toxic if you eat something when your nutritional power is weak. However, if you have the power to turn food into nutrition, even a glass of water can energize you.

Some people believe that it's a sign of good health to be able to eat anything you like as much as you want, but this is really a sign that either your nerves or your internal organs are weak.

The concepts pertaining to prana, which I discussed earlier, can also be applied to food. There are three kinds of nutrition. One is food, and the others are oxygen and internal secretions. If you don't take in as much oxygen as possible, you can't digest your food. If you don't have secretions, you can't absorb your food. Secretions are a medicine within our body that are there to protect our life.

In the yogic concept of food, to absorb nutrition is to connect yourself with the universe through eating and breathing. It's a holy ceremony in which you take other lives as an offering to your life, in order to make the most of yourself. To live is to absorb the energy of the universe using yourself as a medium by moving and thinking. Food, therefore, is the energy of the universe (such as sunshine and air) and the energy of the earth (such as water and minerals) converted.

Elimination is more important than meals

Most people make the mistake of overeating. Many diseases could be cured by correcting this problem. From this viewpoint, modern science is based on convenient reasoning, but not on truth.

Food is absorbed as nutrition most effectively when digestion, respiration, neutralization, and elimination are at a peak. That's why you should eat when you're in good condition to do so, when food tastes good to you. It's also important to vary what you eat in order to stimulate your body. According to yogic principle, you should eat little, but in variety. Foods can be categorized into primary foods, which you can eat throughout the year, and secondary foods, which you should eat only at certain times to stimulate your body.

It's also important to balance ingestion and elimination. If you focus just on eating and neglect elimination, the leftover energy that your body doesn't need will grow. Diseases don't occur due to lack of energy or vitality; rather, our body uses excess energy and vitality to create disease. Eat only once you've completely eliminated what you previously ate. In our yoga dojo, we eat only miso soup for breakfast, and we jog and practice yoga postures to empty our stomach before we eat a real meal for lunch.

I also recommend one minute of meditation before meals. If you eat while you're still excited or tense after work or study, you may end up eating things you don't need. Listen to your body to find out what you want to eat and how hungry you are.

What, how, and how much to eat to be healthy

Your life is determined to a great extent by what and how you eat, because what you eat creates blood, body fluid, muscles, bones – in other words, your body. Since food is related to mind, certain foods can calm or excite us, strengthen or weaken us, and make us more vulnerable or affectionate.

Unfortunately, though, one food is not good for everyone. Each individual has something different that is good, appropriate, and necessary for their body. Vegetarians and natural food types say brown rice is good, but even though it's a good food, eating it all the time can be harmful to some people.

Brown rice is rich in magnesium and tends to destroy calcium, which supports our bones. When you eat brown rice, it's best to sprinkle gomashio (salt and sesame seeds) to balance the minerals.

If there's one principle that applies to everyone, it's this: Enjoy hunger more than fullness. Eat a little of whatever suits your body. You can only find out what's good for your body by observing your hunger.

So how can you find out which foods suit you and your needs? Here are three keys:

①Eliminate bad eating habits by fasting or eating natural foods. Fasting should be done at a retreat with trained instructors. I'll discuss natural foods in more detail later.

②Correct your mistaken ideas about food. I'll discuss this in more detail later as well. To increase the effectiveness of what you eat, use the most healthful cooking methods and combinations of foods.

③Until you find yourself naturally craving foods that are healthy for you, control your diet intentionally. Once you've mastered this, you will naturally sense the correct things to eat, how much to eat, when to eat, and how to eat each day.

The balance of ingredients is important in the yogic way of cooking

In cooking, it's important to balance the characteristics and nutrients of the ingredients you use, without losing these qualities. In other words:

①*Whole foods:* Eat everything together—roots and leaves, peels or rinds, and the flesh of fruits. Natural foods are balanced as a whole.

②*Reuniting way of eating:* Eat both tofu and okara (the soybean fibers left over after making tofu). You should not eat just one part of the soy bean.

③*Blended way of eating:* When you cook meat, include nutrient-rich parts such as the bone and skin.

To heighten the nutritional power of your food, pay attention to the following:

①*Combine foods:* Adding soy beans to rice gives you as much protein as milk. Adding soy to wheat increases essential amino acids. Rice and wheat together combine Yin and Yang. Combining animal protein and plant protein, or animal fat and plant fat, or vegetables and seaweed eliminates any harmful qualities these ingredients contain on their own and raises their nutritional value. The number of calories in many foods increases when they're cooked in oil. The worst example of this is white sugar. Added to foods, it destroys valuable minerals, amino acids, and vitamins.

②*Eat raw foods, primarily vegetables:* Eating raw foods enables you to take in vegetable hormones, vitamins, minerals, and water in their live state. Eating live foods activates the stomach, making it easier to digest other foods, and the abundance of fiber in raw food supports elimination, which prevents fat from accumulating. Eating raw foods also helps your nerves and hormones function in a natural state.

③*Eat dried food:* The minerals, vitamins, and protein in dried foods are more effective because of the sunlight they've absorbed. Dried squid, for example, has five times more protein than fresh squid, as well as more calcium. Dried food also helps cleanse and detoxify. That's why herbal medicines are usually dried.

The following principles of food combination help promote an optimally balanced diet:

A. *Animal protein and plant protein:* Animal protein provides three times more essential amino acids than rice and fifteen times more than potatoes. Vegetable protein contains substances that help you digest, neutralize, and eliminate animal protein.

B. *Animal fat and vegetable fat:* Plant-based fat contains an abundance of essential fatty acid and prevents the build-up of cholesterol from animal fat.

C. *Vegetables, seaweed, bones, and salt:* The human body is healthier when it contains more calcium and natrium magnesium and potassium. Vegetables have a lot of potassium and magnesium, so they should be balanced with bones and salt. If there's too much magnesium and potassium, nerve function will become abnormal.

D. *Seaweed and plant-based vinegar:* The iodine in seaweed increases your ability to burn fat. Adding plant-based vinegar enhances the effect. However, the effect is decreased when combined with too much salt.

E. *Starch and vitamins:* This combination should only be eaten when combined with exposure to sunlight, so it's good for meals in the spring or summer, or at lunchtime.

F. *Animal protein and plant-based acids and minerals:* These are good for meals in the fall and winter, or at dinnertime. The most effective proportion is one part animal to four parts plant.

G. *Calcium and natural sugar:* These provide nutrition for the brain.

However, the effect is eliminated when they're combined with white sugar.

H. *Iron and fruits:* These eliminate toxic gas inside the body. However, the effect is eliminated when iron is combined with too much salt.

I. *Products of the sea and products of the land:* These enhance each other's power and eliminate their negative qualities. Examples include red beans with kelp, or sashimi with fresh vegetables.

Steaming is the best way to cook

In cooking we grind, slice, stew, or grill in order to loosen the molecular bonds in foods, making it easier to combine and balance nutrients and digestive enzyme. The nutritional value of food differs depending on how you heat it, how you add water or condiments, and how you combine different substances.

Steaming is the most efficient way to cook without losing nutrients. Steamed food retains its moisture and is easy to digest. Foods retain most of their nutrients after they're steamed.

The next-best method is stir-frying. Stir-frying with oil increases calories and reduces harmful sugar in foods. Foods that have been stir-fried remain in the stomach for a while working on the stomach wall, so they're full of stamina. (My definition of food with stamina is food that takes longer to digest but that doesn't deprive your body of nutrients, meaning it's safe to store in the body.)

When you cook, don't use much water. Cooking rice with too much water turns it to starch, which is hard to digest. So feeding sick people rice porridge or soup with rice is a misguided idea; it's like feeding them uncooked rice. Dry foods like hardtack contain a better-quality starch.

Meat can't be neutralized unless it's eaten with the bones and skin

Food can be categorized as either acidic or alkaline. The human body is most healthy when it's slightly alkaline, but 80% of Japanese food is excessively acidic. When you're overly acidic, your nerves are tense and your metabolism abnormal, making you tired mentally and physically.

Being too acidic can make children aggressive and adults overly worried or angry. They may get sick easily as well.

Acidic foods include the flesh of all fowl, cattle, and fish; grains;

cocoa; chocolate; alcohol; sugar; and sweets that contain sugar.

Eating alkaline foods neutralizes and eliminates the acidic toxin. Alkaline foods include the bones and skin of fowl, cattle, and fish; raw vegetables; seaweed; sprouts; mushrooms; fruit; and dairy.

But how to best change your intake of acidic or alkaline food depends on your condition.

Eat alkaline foods under the following conditions: when descending a mountain, after crying, after sports, in a noisy place, when you're anxious, when you're angry, after eating meat, after getting cold (especially after swimming), when you do movements that strain your spine, and so on.

Eat acidic food under the following conditions: when ascending a mountain, after laughing, after eating boiled vegetables, in a quiet place, after a break, after warming up (especially after a bath), when you tighten your stomach, and so on.

Food can be categorized as Yin or Yang

All things in the universe are supported by two opposing forces, Yin and Yang. There are Yin and Yang regions, environments, weather, and seasons. Nature is very well thought out: in Yin regions, Yang food is considered healthy, and in Yang seasons, Yin plants grow.

For example, in the hot summer, you may crave foods that cool your body, and in the cold winter, you may crave foods that warm you. Japanese and Europeans have different preference for food because of the difference in Yin and Yang in their environments. Eating vegetables when they're in season is better for your health and balance, so eating seasonal foods makes good sense.

To maintain the balance of humans, animals, and plants, nature provides what's appropriate at the right time and in the right place. Since summer is a Yang season, Yin vegetables grow.

Yin vegetables contain more water to cool the body and promote urination. They're often moist inside, such as tomatoes and watermelons.

In winter, a Yin season, Yang vegetables grow, which warm our body and promote perspiration. These include pumpkins, carrots, mandarin oranges, buckwheat, and other dense vegetables.

But the properties of a vegetable can change depending on its condition. Watery vegetables are Yin when raw but become Yang when dried. The more Yang a food is, the better it is for blood circulation and warming the body.

If you peel a fruit and eat only its flesh, you're just eating the Yin part of the fruit. The skin is Yang. Roots are more Yang than leaves. That's why carrots and lotus roots are good for people who are sick, when the body is more Yin. If a vegetable has a greater ability to receive and absorb sunshine, it's Yang.

You can also be Yin or Yang based on the type of foods you normally eat. Vegetarians are usually Yin. If they eat fruit in addition to all the vegetables they eat, they can become too Yin to be healthy. But if a carnivorous person eats fruit, they can effectively balance Yin and Yang.

A glass of beer after a bath is great because your body is Yang after warming up in the bath, and beer, a Yin drink, balances it.

Because the Yin and Yang of food is relative, you can't always tell what's Yin and what's Yang. Let me give you some common examples.

A. *Umeboshi* (sour pickled plums) and *takuwan* (pickled daikon radish) are *Yan*. Foods become more *Yan* when you reduce the moisture, dry them, heat them, or add salt to them.

B. Rice is *Yang* and wheat is *Yin*. Wheat has less ability to absorb light, so it helps cool us in the summer. That's why straw hats cool the head. Rice and *soba* (buckwheat noodle) are more popular in colder regions because they warm the body.

C. Tuna and sardines are *Yin*, and eel and carp are *Yang*. That's why carp and soft-shelled turtle are good for people who are sick. Soft-shelled turtles have a strong ability to absorb sunshine. Creatures that live underground are even better at this; that's why dried earthworms, for example, are used to treat perspiration.

D. Spicy food is *Yin*, and bitter food is *Yang*. The more expanding the flavor, the more *Yin,* and the less expanding the flavor, the more *Yang*. You could arrange the flavors as follows, from more Yin to Yang: spicy, sour, sweet, salty, bitter.

E. Red food is *Yang*, green is neutral, and white is *Yin*. Carrots are Yang, and eggplants are *Yin*.

We enjoy eating greens in the spring because eating greens that have absorbed so much sunlight neutralizes the excessively Yin foods we consume in the winter. This helps us treat problems such as toxins from animal-based foods, lack of exposure to the sun, and accumulated stool. We should always be grateful for this blessing from nature.

Ying Food
grows in cool dry soil and cold climate
grows slowly hard and contain less moisture

YING and YANG

● take as main items   ● subsidiary items   □ take sometimes   ★ seldam or sometim

▼ Ying ⟵   ⟵ MIDDL

ULTRAVIOLET RAY	PURPLE	INDIGO	BLUE	GREEN
PUNGENT	HOT SPICY	SOUR		SWEET

WATER / CENTRIFUGAL FORCE / POTASSIUM-RICH

grains
□Grain	□Rice Cake	●Brown rice
	□Maize	
	□Wheat noodle	
□Corn		

vegetabls& wild flowers

(eggplants)	(potatoes)	(leaves)	
□Eggplant	□Aroid ⊚Scallion	⊚Japanese raddish	⊚C
■Tomato	□Bamboo shoot ☆Garlic	⊚Cucumber	
■Shiitake	⊚Dried Shiitake	⊚Chinese cabbage	
■Potato	□Sweet potato	⊚Komatsu-na	
		■Spinach	

fruits
■Banana	□Peach	□Apple
■Fig	□Date plum	□Strawberry
□Pineapple	□Tagelin	
□Melon	□Watermelon	
□Grapes		

spices
☆Wasabi	□Ginger	⊚Barilla
☆Pepper	□Curry	⊚Laver
☆Hot pepper		⊚Kelp

legmes
■Soymilk	⊚To-fu	□Fava bean	⊚Fried bean	⊚Red bean
	□Toasted	□Quail bean	curd	⊚Sesame
	soybean flour	□Natto	⊚Freeze-dried To-fu	
			⊚Ganmodoki	

drinks
■Whiskey □Beer		☆Cassia seed tea
■Soda □Sake		□Black tea
■Coffee	□Green tea	☆Allowroot soup
■Cola		●Buckwheat tea
■Brandy		
■Wine		

seasonings / daily products / oil
■White sugar	□Brown sugar	●Sesame oil
■Honey	□Cheese	●Canola oil
■Vinegar	□Milk	□Safflower oil
■MSG	□Yogrut	□Olive oil
	□Peanut butter	

92

FOOD CHART

Yang Food
grows in warm soil and warm climate
grows fast and big with a high water content

as medicines ☐ not neccesary or take very little   ■ take rarely

→⟶ **Yang ▲**

YELLOW	ORANGE	RED		INFRARED RAY
	SALTY		BITTER	ACRID

SODIUM-RICH / CENTRIPETAL FORTH / FIRE

☐Buckwheet noodle
☐Japanese Millet
☐Millet

(root vegetables)
⊚Burdock root   ⊚Japanese Yam
⊚Pumpkin   ⊚Carrot   ☆Dandelion root

⊚Rotus root

(fresh water fish)	(shrimp,crab)	(coast fish)	(deep sea fish)
☐Carp,Eel	☐Flounder	☐Snapper	■ Whale
☐Octopus	☐Trout	☐Sardine	■ Tuna
☐Clam	☐Lobster	☐ Horse mackrel	■ Mackerel
☐Oyster			■ Yellow tail

fish, clams

(moves slowly)   (moves fast)

⊚Seaweed

☐Poultry   ■ Pork
■ Beef
meat   ■ Mutton
☐Egg

● Natural salt   ■ Refined salt
● Soy sauce(used natural&traditional method)
● Bean paste(used natural&tradisional method)
● Pickled plum
● Turnip pickle

Change your diet in summer and winter

In Japan, the four seasons are very distinct, and during each one we see different products in the stores. It's ideal to eat seasonal foods because they taste better, they make sense, and they're good for your body. If you have problem with your appetite because you're too hot or too cold, it's because your body hasn't adapted to the season.

Cells reproduce most often in the spring. Cell reproduction requires fat and protein, which are stored in the winter, as well as activation through glycogen and vitamins, which can be consumed in the spring. We feel dull in the rainy season because our metabolism slows down due to the fat and protein remaining from the winter.

In summer, you perspire more, which causes the blood to be thicker and making it easier to retain heat in the body. During summer, it's best to eat as little as possible, and to eat watery vegetables. If you lack sodium, vitamin B, or vitamin C, you may suffer from heat in the summer. Spicy food is also good because it helps you produce saliva and gastric juices, and contains a lot of vitamin B and C. It's also a good preservative, antibacterial, and vermicide, and supports healthy blood circulation.

Our appetite reaches its peak in the fall. Since the digestive ability is strong then, you can let yourself overeat a little in order to accumulate protein and fat in preparation for winter.

In winter, our body heat dissipates easily. Protein is burned in the liver to warn the body. Plant-based fats are good. It's also important to get enough vitamins.

Food can be medicine, depending how you eat

Medicine is not the only substance that heals diseases. Medicine may be helpful when you're sick, but it can be harmful once you're healed. Therefore, it's safest to do what you can every day to prevent disease. If you think of food as medicine, your meals become the key to your health and hygiene.

Not all foods are medicinal. But if you apply certain tricks to the foods you normally eat, they can help you recover quickly if you do get sick. Here are examples of things you can eat throughout the year:

B. *Pickled vegetables:* These activate your appetite. They contain more nutrients pickled than raw. Since normal pickling methods destroy vitamin C, one trick is to pickle vegetables by adding garlic and red pepper, like with kimchee. Pickling enhances vitamin B_1 and carotene. You can also add seaweed or fish cartilage to supply calcium and iodine. Marinating with miso supplies vitamins A, B, and D. Marinating fish and meat with sake lees or miso makes the bones and skin more palatable and prevents food poisoning.

C. *Soybeans:* These are a high-quality food that contains a lot of protein and fat. Soybeans can prevent arteriosclerosis. However, their nutritional value may change depending on how they're processed. Boiled, only 65% can be digested and absorbed, but if they're processed into tofu, that figure rises to 90%. Tofu also contains calcium. Natto (fermented soybeans) are even more effective, and count as a perfect food. Miso is as good for you as the beans themselves, and eliminates cholesterol and helps growth and digestion. Soybean sprouts contain a lot of vitamin C, and so help with recovery from fatigue and rejuvenation, as well as containing amino acids, which detoxify the liver.

D. *Other beans:* The sugar in azuki beans (red beans) is high quality and easy to digest, and they contain a lot of starch, vitamin B_1, and B_2. They're effective for constipation because they ferment in the body. Peanuts contain fat, protein, and vitamin B_1. Peas contain sugar and vitamin C. Beans are referred to as the "meat of the field," and are highly nutritious, but not as harmful as meat. High-quality grains such as buckwheat, millet, and barnyard grass are good to eat as well.

E. *Brown rice:* This food contains almost all the nutrients we need for survival, including protein, fat, starch, organophosphates, various vitamins, iron, calcium, and manganese. Its protein is the easiest of all foods to absorb and its fat doesn't cause arteriosclerosis. Organophosphates correct imbalances in the blood and nerves. Iron is a nutrient for the blood, and manganese is a nutrient for blood cells. Calcium strengthens our resistance, vitamin A prevents night blindness, vitamin D prevents cavities, and vitamin E prevents sterility. When you eat brown rice, you feel full after eating only one-third as much as white rice, so it doesn't burden your stomach. It can also treat non-disease-related symptoms such as dullness, sleepiness, fatigue, stiffness, flush, cold, and forgetfulness, all of which are caused by eating too much white rice and white bread. Switching from white rice to brown also helps you lose weight because it helps eliminate unnecessary substances from your body. But it's not good to eat too much brown rice. Too much magnesium can hinder muscle strength and the combustion process of cells, which can interfere with your ability to metabolize cholesterol. To prevent this, sprinkle gomashio (salt with sesame) on your rice, because sesame reduces cholesterol.

Even though you know these foods are good for you, it can be hard to change your diet all at once. If that's the case, start by alternating your regular diet with different cooking methods or combinations. Eating brown rice and soy beans will solve most of your physical and mental problems and secure your health for a long time.

I'll now introduce diets that can help you recover from specific problems.

Foods that solve specific problems and difficulties

To enhance brain power: In order to be a quick thinker, you first need sufficient oxygen and glucose, sufficient vitamins to help burn them, and good protein to help the process. Sodium and calcium are needed as well in order to completely neutralize and eliminate unwanted substances such as carbon dioxide, lactic acid, and ammonia. Foods that help with this process include beans, scallions, greens, fruit, egg yolk, liver, butter, cheese, and tomatoes.

The more you use your brain, the better its function will be. Factors that slow the brain include bad blood circulation, lack of oxygen, constant tension, bad posture, and long-term malnutrition.

It's important to avoid overeating and constipation. The less you eat, the better your brain function, and the less tired you'll be.

To enhance beauty: Reduce acidic foods and eat more vegetables, fruit, and seaweed, which are alkaline and contain a lot of vitamins. Calcium is very effective because it cleanses the blood. Vitamins A and D protect the skin, vitamin B improves blood circulation and nerve function, and vitamin C firms the skin and prevents it from darkening.

To lose weight: Don't eat excessive amounts of animal fat, which is highly osmotic, or starch, which turns to fat. (If you want to gain weight, on the other hand, stop eating an unbalanced diet to enhance your ability to absorb nutrients.)

Eat root vegetables, dried vegetables, and seaweed. The iodine in seaweed works to completely burn fat. If you have high blood pressure, eat seaweed with nectar, such as fruit juice, or vinegar. If you're seriously obese, eat a lot of vegetables with minerals and vitamins and only a small amount of plant-based fat.

To grow taller: You need calcium and vitamins. As for food, small fish, carrots, and cabbage are good choices.

For beautiful skin: Your sweat needs to be alkaline – acidic sweat causes the skin to deteriorate. As for food, apples, celery, and parsley are good choices.

For pregnancy and an easy delivery: It's said that you can choose your baby's gender by changing the constitution of your blood, and that if you take a lot of calcium you're more likely to have a boy.

Pregnancy depletes the mother's vitamins, calcium, iron, and other minerals, so you need to be cautious with nutrition. A nutritional imbalance can cause miscarriage.

Overeating is not healthy. Because the stomach is related to the sex organs, you may experience more morning sickness and changes of appetite if your stomach is weak.

During pregnancy don't eat too much starch; get more of your calories from fat; and eat foods high in protein, vitamin A, B vitamins, calcium, and iron. But salt and water can cause swelling. Eating too much sugar, fruit, starch, and animal products make you more likely to have a difficult delivery.

For irregular menstruation: Eat foods containing vitamin B, vitamin C, calcium, and sodium. Eating macro-vegetarian food is effective, especially a lot of root vegetables and seaweed.

For better sex: The nerves that control appetite and sex drive are located in the same area of the brain – so if your diet is wrong, your sexual ability can be affected. For example, a lack of vitamins and excess blood sugar can lower your ability to be aroused. Overeating can numb the nerves.

Impotence and frigidity can be treated with foods that contain the type of good protein necessary for proper functioning of the adrenal gland and other hormonal glands. These include beans, meat, eggs, milk, healthy types of fat, and vitamins B, C, K, and E. Stimulants such as garlic, onion, red pepper, carrots, and ginger are also very effective. Constipation diminishes arousal because it lessens abdominal muscle pressure.

For headache: Eat whole foods and raw vegetables for sufficient calcium and vitamin B_1. Small fish, seaweed, lotus root, carrots, celery, red beans, sesame, green tea, and daikon radish are all effective.

For insomnia: Good choices include brown rice, dark bread, vegetables, seaweed, small fish, beans, lotus root, onion, carrots, and pumpkin.

For nearsightedness and astigmatism: Make sure you're getting enough vitamins A, B, C, and calcium. Alkaline food such as vegetables, seaweed, and fruit are good, but limit your intake of meat, eggs, fish, butter, and cheese, all of which oxidize the blood.

For ear and nose problems: Take calcium and vitamins B and C. Brown rice and dark bread are also effective. Eat raw vegetables if your body type is Yang, and stir-fried vegetables if your body type is Yin.

For stiff shoulders and neck: Eat brown rice, vegetables, seaweed, beans, daikon radish, konnyaku (alimentary yam paste), and hijiki (seaweed).

For asthma: Foods that contain vitamin B and C are helpful. Too much starch makes you constipated, which causes gas to travel up the body and increases coughing. Protein creates phlegm, so limit it to as little as possible. Lotus root, black beans, pumpkin, onion, carrots, comfrey, and seaweed are good choices.

To strengthen the internal organs: Vitamins, calcium, and sodium are important, as are good vegetable nutrients and good protein. Adlai (a corn-like grain), black sesame seeds, black beans, snails, pine needles, garlic, walnuts, scallions, onion, eels, sprouts, and yams are good.

Organ prolapse: Avoid overeating and the use of toxic substances, and eat foods with lots of Yang-type minerals such as calcium, sodium, and iron. Note that if you eat too much meat or starchy food, you will never get a sufficient amount of minerals.

Because organ prolapse and apathy are Yin Kyosho (a sickness caused by the degeneration or lack of seiki, a concept in Chinese medicine that is close to the idea of immune system), you should avoid sugar and fruit, and instead eat brown rice, burdock, carrots, natto (fermented soy), hijiki (seaweed), kombu kelp, small fish, black sesame seeds, and scallions.

Back pain: Eat foods that are high in vitamins B and C, calcium, and sodium, and avoid too much sugar and animal fat. Macro-vegetarian foods are good, especially root vegetables and seaweed.

Constipation: Brown rice, fiber-rich vegetables, seaweed, and pickles are good, especially burdock, konnyaku, Japanese yams, daikon radish, hijiki, kombu kelp, wakame (seaweed), and natto.

Chapter 3

Strengthening the Body and Mind

1. TO ENHANCE BEAUTY AND INTELLIGENCE

Yoga for everyday problems

Now that I've introduced some methods to improve your body and mind as a whole, I'd like to offer my solutions for dealing with particular worries, bad habits, and minor illnesses.

As you read through these, you may think they're too easy, or even silly. But they're all very effective. Modern people don't bother doing even these simple things – in part because our lifestyle makes it difficult for us to do things that are good for our body.

For example, if you study in school or work at a desk for a long time, your brain slows down and you become inefficient. The best solution is to yawn, which circulates blood through your body and brain – but this may be difficult to do if it's considered inappropriate to yawn in class or at work.

When animals find themselves like this, they stretch or yawn to correct their body, so they don't end up with headache later on like humans do.

The best thing for your body to do in this state is to stand up and stretch. In yoga, we also recommend putting pressure on the temples with your fists. Tightening the skull is a very effective way to improve blood circulation.

Interlace your hands behind your neck and arch your back with your chin pointing to the ceiling, bending your neck back as much as possible. Grabbing and rotating your feet also improves blood circulation to the brain. You can do these exercises easily during a break. They will definitely improve your efficiency.

You may want to lose weight or be smarter, you may feel dull, suffer from insomnia, have an upset stomach, or your skin may look dull. Or you may be apathetic, unable to focus on work, or blush when you see someone. You may have countless problems – but you're making your life even more miserable by thinking of those problems all the time. Let's fix them all with yoga right now.

What we do from now on determines whether we're humans or just animals. Animals live merely to exist, but humans live to live life. Animals know how to deal with diseases and problems on their own to survive. In the past, humans also possessed this ability, but now it has become weak.

We've lost the ability to live the way we are, but we still have the ability to make the most of life. We can live the life we want.

If you have minor problems in your life, you can deal with them using the following techniques.

Headache: Before deciding to take medication, try putting on a headband or cooling your head to tighten the skull and improve blood circulation. Often one side of the skull is lower than the other, so have someone check if one ear is lower. Lightly pound the back of the ear that's lower with a fist, bottom to top. This treats congestion in the brain and clears the mind.

Lack of sleep: Bend your neck and look down so that the back of your head faces up, and pound it lightly with your fists. When you're sleepy, you might also try stretching and flexing with your legs open wide, like sumo wrestlers do.

Insomnia: Do stretching poses to stretch the whole body. Stretching the muscles relaxes them.

For good sleep: Your mattress should be firm and your pillows thin. Once you're in bed, relax your muscles by thinking of some happy childhood memories. Yogis have practiced this technique for thousands of years.

To strengthen your intellect:

A. Do a headstand. Your mind becomes clouded when the blood circulation in your brain is poor. When you stand on your head, fresh blood travels there.
B. Put on a headband. Cool your head and tighten your skull for better blood circulation.
C. Study on a relatively empty stomach. Sit on a firm chair and keep your spine straight.
D. Pound your coccyx with your fists to send more blood to the brain.

E. Massage your head with your fists. Move from the temples to the forehead, side of the head, back of the head, and top of the head. Light pounding is very effective as well. It's the easiest way to relax a tired brain. For greater effectiveness, try it after a warm bath.

When your head is tired: Open your chest and interlace your fingers behind your back. Then stretch your arms behind your back, with your palms facing out. You might want to stretch the Achilles tendons as well. Simply rotating the ankles can be effective.

To prevent dandruff: Dandruff occurs when you're too acidic or eat too much Yang food. It's also related to malnutrition and anxiety. Washing the hair too often is not good either.

To prevent gray hair: Hairs often turns gray due to stress, worry, serious disease, sudden fear, and other reasons. When our hair turns gray, our scalp is loose and inactive. The solution is to improve blood circulation in the scalp. Supported Headstand Pose (Salamba Sirsasana), Supported Shoulderstand Pose (Salamba Sarvangasana), and Twisting Pose are effective.

To prevent baldness: Baldness occurs when the scalp gets hard and blocks the blood circulation, resulting in malnutrition. Supported Headstand Pose (Salamba Sirsasana) and Supported Shoulderstand Pose (Salamba Sarvangasana) help tighten the scalp and improve blood circulation. If your lower back is weak, you're more likely to be bald.

For nearsightedness:

A. Hold your right earlobe with your left hand, and your left earlobe with your right hand. Pull down on your earlobes as you exhale in short, forceful repetitions. Tighten your stomach as you exhale. The ears contain acupuncture points for the eyes.

B. Move your eyeballs up and down, right and left, and then diagonally. Or try going back and forth between looking at something in the distance and something close by. When you're nearsighted, your eye muscles are contracted, so look at something in the distance as often as possible to stretch the muscles.

C. Stimulate the indentations on the back of your head, just behind the eyes, by massaging the points with your thumbs.

For eye fatigue: Sit in seiza and interlace your fingers behind your back. Bend your upper body forward as you exhale and shut your eyes tight while you pull your hands up toward the ceiling.

For dizziness: Standing up quickly can cause anemia in the brain because our blood pressure is different when we're sleeping or sitting than when we're standing. This is usually caused by a physical condition, so try to keep your body healthy. Bathing in cold water in the summer helps the blood vessels contract.

For tinnitus and hearing problems: This is caused by stiffness of the neck muscles and the muscles in the back of the legs.
   A. Repeatedly bend your neck to the left as you inhale, then to the right as you exhale. Repeat the reverse. Pounding the base of the neck is also helpful.
   B. Practice *Aodake-fumi* (step over a piece of fresh bamboo, split in half, two feet long and five inches in diameter, with the cut side toward the floor, or step on glass bottles (such as Coke bottles) to soften the muscles on the bottom of the feet.

For emphysema:
   A. Holding your jaw tightly closed, try to open your mouth against the pressure. Repeat. Massage the side of the nose from the bottom up.
   B. Switch to a diet made up of small portions, primarily vegetables.
   C. Tuck in your chin and arch your back.

For bad breath: While this can be caused by cavities, it usually occurs when food in the stomach and intestines ferments in an unusual way. Eat plenty of raw vegetables and drink water with minerals.

For teeth grinding: Treat your stiff neck and body distortion and wear thin, light clothing. Bathing in cold water is effective as well.

For snoring: The primary causes of snoring are distortion of the neck and lower back. Remove the snorer's pillow or shake their body. When their neck is straight, they'll stop snoring.

For acne: Skin is closely related to your mental state, so when you're happy your skin looks beautiful. The amount and content of your food also greatly affects your skin. Avoid sweets and be careful to eat a balanced diet. Body distortion can be another cause. For example, if your body is tilted forward somewhat, you'll suffer from acne on your forehead and below your mouth. If your body is weighted to one side, you'll have acne on that side. If your body is twisted, you'll have acne on your cheeks. And if your center of gravity is not low enough, you probably have acne around your mouth.

For stiff shoulders and neck: Suffering from chronic stiff shoulders or neck doesn't necessarily mean that just your shoulders and neck are tired. This problem is caused by a build-up of various factors such as nervousness, mental fatigue, malfunction of the organs or the blood pressure, malnutrition, and bad posture.

A. Stretch your arms to the side, parallel to the floor, and twist them forward and backward as if you were rolling your hands and arms. Repeat this twisting motion while holding your arms to the front, to the back, to the sky, and to the ground.

B. Practice Supported Headstand Pose (*Salamba Sirsasana*), Supported Shoulderstand Pose (*Salamba Sarvangasana*), or Plow Pose and six repetitions of abdominal breathing.

For beautifully shaped shoulders: If one of your shoulders is higher than the other, or if the tops of your shoulders aren't parallel to the floor, you have bad posture. If you usually carry a shoulder bag on one side, switch to the other. If you're right-handed, you probably carry a bag on your right shoulder, so that side will tend to be higher. Carry your bag on your left shoulder until the problem is fixed.

For tired hands and arms: The hands are closely related to the brain and the internal organs. If one of your fingers is bent, stiff, or cold, it's a sign that the nerves or organs connected to that finger has a problem. Conversely, a problem with your finger can cause your internal organs to malfunction. Modern diseases such as a carpal tunnel syndrome are a phenomenon caused by overuse of the fingers.

A. If your right hand or arm is tired, balance both sides by using your left hand and arm. This is much more effective than massaging the tired arm. Doing the same movements on the opposite side can correct imbalance and distortion and help reduce the problem. In addition, try to relax your left hand when you use your right one.

B. Release excess energy from your hands and shoulders when you work or study. Stiffness in the hands and tension in the brain are related. If you tend to use a lot of pressure when you write, learn to use a mechanical pen, which requires less pressure and will teach you to relax your hand.

For slim, beautiful wrists: Do push-ups, variously pointing your fingers front, back, left, and right. Do more repetitions of whichever version is most difficult.

For slim arms: When your breathing power is weak, your arms become weaker. This weakness in the arms can cause visceroptosis or splanchnoptosis, a prolapse or sinking of the abdominal viscera below their natural position. Any or all organs may be displaced downward. When the intestines are involved, the condition is known as enteroptosis; when the stomach is found below its normal position, the term gastroptosis is used. This disease exists in all degrees of severity and may give rise to no symptoms whatsoever. It can also cause costa descensus, an abnormal downward bending of the ribs that can coincide with visceroptosis (though not vice versa). Try to lift and lower your arms as you twist and rotate your wrists.

For frostbite: Wearing something thin toughens your skin and helps you get used to the cold weather, as does bathing in cold water followed immediately by hot – even during the summer. If you have frostbite, soak your hands in warm salt water. Once they're warm, switch to cold water. Repeat.

For a cold: Colds are caused by an imbalanced diet. It's important to change your diet, especially if you're overeating and nutritionally imbalanced. When you have a cold, your muscles become contracted and tense. Move your body to relax your muscles and promote sweating, then dry your body well and go to sleep quietly. Coughing or sneezing intentionally causes your body temperature to rise and your body to relax.

To reduce the harmful effects of smoking: Smoke different types of cigarettes. If you smoke the same brand all the time, you become accustomed to the same stimuli and will eventually have to increase the amount you smoke in order to achieve the same level of stimulation. Taking the same kind of stimulants all the time doesn't enhance your ability to adapt.

For breast enhancement: Stand with your back straight and your hips tight. Place your hands under your ribcage and bend your neck backward. Then lift your ribs as you inhale deeply. Hold your breath as long as possible, then bend forward slightly, crossing your arms in front of you as you exhale completely.

For motion sickness: Motion sickness is caused by a crooked, stiff neck. Stretch your neck to the side opposite the one it's bent toward, and rotate your head to increase flexibility.

To increase or decrease appetite: Lack of appetite is your body's natural reaction to something, so don't force yourself to eat. You can make your stomach more active by arching your back. To avoid overeating, control your stomach's activity by pressing or tapping your forehead lightly with your palms.

For stomachache due to overeating: Bend forward as far as possible as you exhale forcefully. Hold your breath for a while in this position, then arch your back as you inhale. Repeat. If one of your legs is shorter than the other, stretch the shorter leg.

To reduce the harmful effects of drinking: Drink only when you're happy. There's nothing more harmful than drinking to escape worries or deal with stress.

A. If you're sitting down while you're drinking, rotate one of your ankles while keeping your toes on the floor to help remove alcohol from your body. It's also a good idea to alternate drinking water and alcohol.

B. Interlace your fingers behind your neck, tuck in your chin, and push your head up forcefully with your hands.

For hangover: Hold your arms out to the side, parallel to the floor, and bend your elbows so that your lower arms point to the ceiling. Make fists. Twist your upper body left and right as you exhale slowly, imagining that you're exhaling all the alcohol, as if you could light a fire with your breath. Relax and return to center. Lightly pound the back of your head. You can also do this while you're drinking.

For a strong stomach: Our stomach is deeply related to our senses. In fact, people have believed that our kokoro (heart/mind) is in our chest. That's because our inner psychology or feelings appear directly in our stomach or heart. If you're worried or stressed for a while, your stomach will get sick.

Laugh from your heart at least once a day. Strengthen your mind so that things don't affect you as easily, and learn to laugh at little things. Stretching the left side of your body will help as well.

For constipation:

A. Drink cold water – one cup of thin salt water before bed, and another half cup of salt water with a half cup of cold water when you get up. Alternatively, you can drink a cup of lukewarm water (70% cold water and 30% hot water). But don't drink too much.

B. When you're constipated, your right arm is stiff. Massage it to eliminate stiffness.

C. Rub your left palm with your right middle finger (acupressure points for the intestines are on the left palm).

D. Upon awakening, bend your knees and straighten them toward the ceiling as you massage your stomach with circular movements.

For diarrhea: Diarrhea is the body's own effort to eliminate toxins, so it's best to cooperate with your body. Shaking your hips like a hula or disco dancer is good for diarrhea because it relaxes the hips and contracts the buttocks.

For hemorrhoids: Hemorrhoids can only be cured through anal surgery. Even if you think you're cured, you will have another breakout. Hemorrhoids are a whole-body problem caused by looseness in the intestines. This means that you need to improve your lifestyle by changing your diet, posture, and breath.

A. Walk with weights on your big toes. Massage your little toes thoroughly when you wake up or after you bathe.
B. Stand on one foot. This builds strength in the legs and buttocks and contracts the sphincter muscle.

For menstrual problems: People often say you should rest and avoid playing sports or taking baths during menstruation, but that's all superstition. Changes in the body are natural during menstruation. Get plenty of exercise before menstruation. Eliminate body distortion. Menstrual pain will decrease if you stop eating too much sugar and animal products.

For morning sickness: This is caused by the inability of the pelvis to open and close. Push your knees open on both sides to stretch.

For more powerful sex:
A. Sit in seiza, tighten your sphincter, and lift your body. Strengthening the sphincter muscle also strengthens the sex organs.
B. Walk with strength in your big toes to make your ankle and legs stronger. If your legs are big or bowed, your sexual ability will tend to be low.
C. Exercise a lot and keep your muscles flexible, so that they have the ability to contract and relax easily. If you don't exercise, your muscles get tense and lose their elasticity. When your body can contract and relax flexibly, your sexual pleasure is enhanced.
D. Put more force on your exhalation than on your inhalation, and hold your breath for as long as possible. If you exhalation is

longer and stronger, you'll increase your activity level and vitality, and if you can hold your breath longer, you'll be able to contract with more force.

To enhance sexual pleasure: People's capacity for sexual pleasure varies at different stages, and varies greatly from person to person. In general, women need to be relaxed at the beginning of a sexual encounter in order to contract when necessary. It takes them a while to relax after intercourse as well. In short, they need sufficient foreplay and loving touch. On the other hand, men are contracted right from the beginning and release quickly. The best way to cure frigidity or premature ejaculation is to match your rhythm with your partner's. Sexual pleasure is release from desire (tension), therefore it's helpful to practice focusing and relaxing repeatedly in your daily life.

To reduce sex drive: Using both hands to hold your knees tightly together, try to open them. Follow by rotating your hips and neck to relax and taking some deep breaths.

To prevent your feet from falling asleep: Stretch your hips, ankles, and Achilles tendons. To make your legs and feet less apt to fall asleep, keep one big toe on top of the other while sitting in seiza, switching them around every several minutes.

For slender hips: Slender hips are not only beautiful, they're also the basis for being able to move quickly. Keep your feet shoulder-width apart, hands on the hips, and draw a figure eight with your hips as you exhale.

For tired legs: Your legs are more likely to get tired if you're tilted forward, which contracts the Achilles tendons. Fix your posture, keep your strength on your big toes, and walk rhythmically. Practice walking backward. Slide backward, keeping your feet on the ground. Humans usually walk forward, but doing the opposite can help you recover from fatigue. Using muscles that don't usually get much use helps your legs become stronger and less tired.

For athlete's foot: Massage the troubled area. The major cause of athlete's foot is lack of blood circulation in the area, so massage or rotate each toe when you get up and before you go to sleep.

To beautify the legs and slim the ankles: Stand on tiptoe at the edge of the stairs or a threshold, keeping your weight on your toes. Lift and lower your body using only the strength of your lower legs. Inhale as you lift and exhale as you lower. Repeat thirty times.

When your feet fall asleep: To fix this while remaining seated, lift your buttocks slightly and repeatedly tighten and relax your whole legs. If you can stand up, walk backward, sliding your feet on the floor.

For fatigue: Lie down and lift your right leg perpendicular to the floor. Massage your leg from ankle to thigh as if squeezing a wet cloth. Repeat on the left leg. Continue until the fatigue disappears. Doing this before a bath increases its effectiveness.

For hunger, thirst, sleepiness, or laziness: Practice frog breathing technique. Curl your tongue so that the tip lightly touches the back of the roof of your mouth. Open your mouth slightly and inhale slowly, making a sound. Breathe in through your mouth and out through your nose. This technique promotes beauty and strengthens the body.

For weight loss:
   A. Sit in seiza. Place your buttocks between your legs and lower your upper body backward to the floor. Grab your ankles with your hands and gently lift your upper body as you exhale. This makes your upper body beautiful, especially the bust line.
   B. Get on all fours, with your toes standing on the floor. Touch the floor with your chest, keeping your hands below your chin. Inhale, and as you exhale tilt your hip to the right. Bring it back to center as you inhale. Don't lift your elbows. Repeat on the left. Repeat these movements as quickly as you can. Do more repetitions on the side that's harder. This exercise slims the entire body.

2. HEALING DISEASE THROUGH ACTIVE POSES

How to self-check your body

In this section, I introduce exercises to restore the body to its natural, healthy state. In contrast to the inactive poses introduced in chapter 1, I refer to these as active poses, or body-correcting exercises.

Before we begin, let's see where you have problems in your body. If you can't do the following movements or postures, you have problems in the corresponding areas of the body.

① Lie on your back with the bottoms of your feet touching. If your knees remain above the floor, you have problems with your pelvis.

② Lie on your back with your hands at your sides. If your knee bends when you lift your leg straight up, you have problems in thoracic vertebra #12, lumbar vertebra #1, and sacral vertebrae #1 and #2; in other words, in one or more upper vertebrae. (These are numbered one through three.

③ Lie on your back, interlace your fingers behind your neck, and twist your upper body from side to side, keeping both shoulders on the floor. If your shoulder lifts, you have problems in thoracic vertebrae #5 and #10.

④ Lie on your back with your legs spread wide. Bend one knee and, keeping your foot on the floor, try to touch the floor between your legs with the bent knee. If your knee doesn't touch the floor, you have problems in lumbar vertebra #3.

⑤ Lie on your back with your legs in Hero Pose (virasana; pose #10) and grab your ankles. If you can't lift your upper body, your stomach and your ability to tighten your pelvis are weak.

⑥ If you can't do Plow Pose (Halasana), you have problems in thoracic vertebrae #1, 2, and 8, and lumber vertabrae #1 and 2.

⑦ Lie on your back, bend your knees, and drop both knees to the same side. If your knees can't touch the floor, you have problems in thoracic vertebrae #10, 11, and 12.

⑧ Lie on your back, hold your knees tight to your chest, and raise yourself to a seated position. If you can't do so, your shoulders are stiff and you have problems in thoracic vertebra #7.

⑨ If you can't tilt you upper body backward from a kneeling position, your pelvis is too tight.

⑩ Sit on the floor with your legs in front of you and practice Sitting Forward Bend Pose (*Paschimottanasana;* see page 30). If your knees bend, you have problems in thoracic vertebra #12 and lumbar vertabra #1.

⑪ If your knees bend when you stand and bend forward, you have problems in lumbar vertebrae #1 and 5.

⑫ Lie on your back, interlace your fingers behind your neck, and begin spreading your legs. If your knees bend and your elbows can't stay on the floor, you have problems with your lower lumbar area and pelvis.

⑬ Sit on the floor with the bottoms of your feet touching. If the tips of your feet can't stay on the floor, you have problems in your sacral area. If your knees can't stay on the floor, you have problems in your organs of elimination.

Each bone mentioned above is related to a separate nerve in a separate part of the body and its organs. If a bone is distorted or dislocated, the related organ will be weak or damaged or nearly to the point of disease. Refer to the diagram in the book for more information.

How the body gets distorted

Why do these kinds of problems happen to the bones? In short, because of bad posture. But we can't always have good posture. We're always straining some part of our body as we stand, walk, or sit down.

When you stand, for example, you work lumbar vertebra #1, which is then more likely to have trouble.

In the same way, a writing job works lumbar vertebra #2, a job that requires sitting in a chair works lumbar vertebra #3, sitting postures work lumbar vertebra #4, sitting in a half-crouch or half-squat (thighs not touching the calves) works thoracic vertebra #10, bending forward works thoracic vertebrae #5 and #6, and a job that requires hand movements such as typing works the cervical vertebrae, making them vulnerable to problems. If these tasks are done for only a few minutes a day, there won't be a problem, but if you stay in the same posture for a long time at work or due to habit, the problem can become entrenched.

Next, I introduce methods that use movement and visual appearance to help you sort out problems.

① Stand, sit, lie on your back, and then lie on your stomach. Observe these inactive postures to find any distortion, crookedness, or imbalance.

The key to correcting these problems is to stretch any areas that are contracted, soften areas of stiffness, and contract stretched areas. As you do so, change direction, speed, and strength according to the strength of your ki or according to how old the problem is, and breathe in a rhythm that feels appropriate.

If a distortion is old a nd severe, contract any contracted areas even further, or if your body is twisted, twist further in that direction. If you're young and healthy, do this quickly and forcefully, as if trying to shock the body.

If the distortion is relatively new and less severe, or if your body is weak due to other diseases or problems, correct it by doing just the opposite. Twist your body in the opposite direction, or stretch the contracted area. If you're old or in poor health, do this as slowly as possible.

② As you do the postures, if you notice a difference in strength between the right and left or front and back of your body, gather force into the weak area, and release force from the stronger area. There is an active technique that draws more force into areas of abundant force, and a passive technique that disperses force to different areas. If one area is weak and lacks force, do a posture that strengthens it, holding the posture for a while to enable you to focus force in that area.

Diagram Showing the Relationship Between the Vertebra and Internal Organs

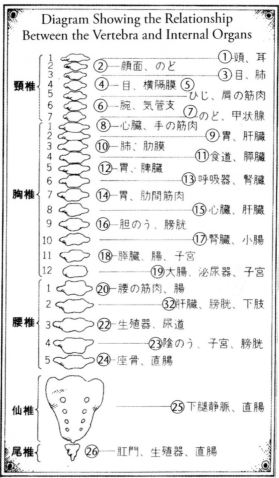

頸椎
- 1
- 2 ②顔面、のど ①頭、耳
- 3 ③目、肺
- 4 ④目、横隔膜 ⑤
- 5 ひじ、肩の筋肉
- 6 ⑥腕、気管支 ⑦のど、甲状腺
- 7

胸椎
- 1 ⑧心臓、手の筋肉
- 2 ⑨胃、肝臓
- 3 ⑩肺、肋膜 ⑪食道、膵臓
- 4
- 5 ⑫胃、脾臓 ⑬呼吸器、腎臓
- 6
- 7 ⑭胃、肋間筋肉
- 8 ⑮心臓、肝臓
- 9 ⑯胆のう、膀胱
- 10 ⑰腎臓、小腸
- 11 ⑱膵臓、腸、子宮
- 12 ⑲大腸、泌尿器、子宮

腰椎
- 1 ⑳腰の筋肉、腸
- 2 ㉜肝臓、膀胱、下肢
- 3 ㉒生殖器、尿道
- 4 ㉓陰のう、子宮、膀胱
- 5 ㉔座骨、直腸

仙椎
- ㉕下腿静脈、直腸

尾椎
- ㉖肛門、生殖器、直腸

① head, ear ② face, throat ③ eye, lung ④ eye, diaphragm ⑤ elbow, muscle of shoulder ⑥ arms, bronchitis ⑦ throat, thyroid ⑧ heart muscle of hands ⑨ stomach, liver ⑩ lung, pleure ⑪ esophagus, pancreas ⑫ stomach, spleen ⑬ respiratory, organs, kidney ⑭ stomach, intercoastals' muscle ⑮ heart, liver ⑯ gallbladder, bladder ⑰ kidney, small intestine ⑱ pancreas, intestine, uterus ⑲ large intestine, urology, uterus ⑳ hip muscle, intestine ㉑ liver, bladder ㉒ genital, urethra ㉓ cod, uterus, bladder ㉔ sciatic, rectum ㉕ lower limb vein, rectum ㉖ anus, genital

Spine exercises

Where were your problems located? Here are some techniques to treat those problems by correcting the spine and stimulating the associated organs.

The human spine is shaped like a spring with a beautiful S-shaped curve. But it becomes dislocated through (1) bad habits, (2) disease, and (3) efforts to protect the body from bad habits and disease. Problems in the organs and spinal nerves distort the backbone, which is directly related to the problem areas. So problems in different parts of the body can be cured by stimulating the spine directly.

The spine consists of twenty-seven parts: the cervical vertebrae (#1 through 7), the thoracic vertebrae (#1 through 12), the lumbar vertebrae (#1 through 5), and the sacral vertebrae (#1 through 3). I'll look at each of these, and discuss how to apply stimulation to them and what results to expect.

This will all take place while lying on your back. Lie down with this book in your hand.

Stimulating the cervical vertebrae

1. *Cervical vertebrae #1 and 2:* To correct the eyes, ears, movement of the blood vessels, and blood circulation to the brain.

   Lie on your back and point your toes up, stretching your Achilles tendons. Lift your chin. Place your hands to your sides, palms facing down. As you exhale, lift your legs, and lower them as you inhale.

2. *Cervical vertebra #3:* For the eyes, ears, nose, throat, and teeth, to stimulate the organs, and to improve blood circulation to the brain.

   Repeat the previous exercise with your chin tucked in.

3. *Cervical vertebra #4:* For the heart, diaphragm, eyes, ears, and nose, and to treat hiccups.

   Repeat the previous exercise to the point where you tuck in your chin. Instead, lift your head and legs without bending your knees as you exhale.

4. *Cervical vertebra #5:* To stimulate the heart, throat, diaphragm, eyes, and ears.

   Keep your legs hip-width apart. Interlace your fingers behind your neck, keep your elbows on the floor, and open your chest. Push against floor with the back of your head and lift your hips.

5. *Cervical vertebra #6:* To stimulate the throat, hands, heart, and thyroid.

   Keep your legs together and stretch your Achilles tendons. Bend your elbows 90 degrees and make fists. Take a deep breath and hold it for one second. As you exhale, tuck in your chin and lift your legs.

6. *Cervical vertebra #6:* To stimulate the throat, heart, vagus nerves, and hands.

   Keep your feet together. Bend your elbows 90 degrees, make fists, and point them at your feet. Take a deep breath and hold it, focusing on and strengthening your tanden. Without releasing the strength, bring force to your elbows. Exhale forcefully as you stretch your Achilles tendons, tuck in your chin, and push against the floor with your hands and elbows. Keep your awareness on the base of your neck. Lift your legs slightly and relax as you exhale.

Stimulating the thoracic vertebrae

1. *Thoracic vertebra #1:* To stimulate the windpipe, heart, and arms.

   Keep your feet hip-width apart. With your hands on your chin, extend your elbows to both sides as far as you can and lift your head. Hold and bear with it for a while, and gently release down.

2. *Thoracic vertebra #2:* For the windpipe, heart, and arms.

   With your feet hip-width apart, hold your head in both hands and lift. Hold for a while and slowly release it down.

3. **Thoracic vertebra #3:** To oppress ((suppress or strengthen?)) the lungs, heart, and vagus nerves.

   With your feet hip-width apart, lift your legs, stretching the Achilles tendons. With your hands on the base of your shoulders, pull your elbows apart.

4. **Thoracic vertebra #4:** To eliminate stiffness in the neck, liver, lungs, and shoulders; to improve blood circulation to the brain.

   With your feet hip-width apart, lift your legs. Bend your elbows 90 degrees, makes fists, and point them at your feet. Exhale forcefully as you stretch your Achilles tendons, tuck in your chin, and push against the floor with your hands and elbows. Slide your elbows toward your head, keeping them on the floor.

5. **Thoracic vertebra #5:** For the throat, eyes, ears, hands, and stomach; to eliminate congestion in the chest and abdominal area; to strengthen the lungs; to treat constipation and obesity; to enhance sex drive; and to balance the nerves and endocrine glands in the brain.

   With your legs hip-width apart, lift your legs. Keep your elbows bent next to the chest, hands up, and arch your back using your chin as you exhale. Stretch your chest and Achilles tendons. (See Fish Pose)

6. **Thoracic vertebra #6:** For the stomach, diaphragm, pleurae, feet, thyroid, and spleen.

   With your feet slightly more than hip-width apart, lift your legs. Lift your hands toward the ceiling and cross your arms while keeping your elbows straight, as if you were hugging something small very tightly.

7. **Thoracic vertebra #7:** For the stomach, diaphragm, and adrenal gland.

   Bend your lower legs to the side (Wariza, or Hero Pose [Virasana]) and grab your ankles. Tuck in your chin and sit up.

8. *Thoracic vertebra #8:* For the plurae, diaphragm, spleen, and liver; to enhance the elasticity of the abdominal area; to stretch the muscles in the front of the thighs; to correct anteflexion, an entrenched forward-bending of the upper body from the waist due to osteoporosis caused by aging.

Practice Wariza (Hero Pose, or Virasana), grab your ankles, and lift up your hips.

9. *Thoracic vertebra #9:* For the spleen, pancreas, and bladder, and to support the sympathetic nerves.

Bend one knee, lean it toward the other leg/knee, and try to touch the floor with it. Interlace your fingers behind your neck and slowly bend your leg right and left, keeping your upper body on the floor. Switch legs and repeat.

10. *Thoracic vertebra #10:* For the eyes, to stretch the muscles of the inner thighs, and to treat the kidneys and uterus.

With your legs together, stretch your Achilles tendons. Push your hands to the front, sit half-way up, and move your hands up and down.

11. *Thoracic vertebra #11:* For the kidneys, uterus, stomach, and intestines, and to correct dislocation of the organs.

Bend your left knee, lean it toward the other leg/knee, and try to touch the floor with the knee (almost like a half-Wariza, or Hero Pose [Virasana]). Grab your left ankle with your left hand and sit up with your right arm stretched. Change legs and repeat.

12. *Thoracic vertebra #12:* To support the large and small intestines and appendix and to contract the stomach, intestines, and liver; to generally strengthen the internal organs.

Open your legs slightly with your arms stretched to the side and your chin tucked in. Stretch your Achilles tendons forcefully, as if you're lifting your feet off the floor so that the heels are not touching the floor, and hold for a while.

Stimulating the lumbar vertebrae

1. *Lumbar vertebra #1:* To contract the eyes, bladder, sex organs, stomach, intestines, and liver and to recover from fatigue.

Stretch your arms out at your sides at shoulder height, with your feet hip-width apart. Stretch your hands and feet and lift your hips as you exhale.

2. *Lumbar vertebra #2:* To contract the stomach and intestines and stimulate the appendix.

Stretch your arms above your head. Keep your feet together and sit up as you exhale.

3. *Lumbar vertebra #3:* To influence the sex organs, legs, and pituitary gland.

With your feet hip-width apart, stretch your arms in front of you and tuck in your chin. Lift your upper body slowly, twist it to the left, and sit up. Repeat to the right.

4. *Lumbar vertebra #4:* To promote elimination and stimulate the sex organs reproductive, large intestines, and legs.

Bend your left leg inward and interlace your hands behind your head. Take a deep breath and hold. Focusing on your abdominal area, move to the right and left as you exhale forcefully, keeping your left knee on the floor.

5. *Lumbar vertebra #5:* For the bladder, sex organs, and blood circulation in the legs.

Placing the bottoms of your feet together, interlace your fingers behind your neck and move your body left and right as you exhale.

Stimulating the sacral vertebrae

1. *Sacral vertebrae #1 and 2:* For the bladder, sex organs, and legs.
2. *Sacral vertebra #3:* To stimulate the sphincter and sex organs.

Bend your knees and, keeping your feet on the floor, lift your hips. Keep your feet slightly apart to stimulate the upper sacral area, wide apart to stimulate the lower sacral area.

These spinal exercises form the base for the active postures I'm about to introduce. Keep in mind what you've just learned by doing the exercises and you'll have a greater understanding of how the postures affect your body.

How to use and practice the thirty-six basic active postures

These basic active postures are also called body-correcting exercises. While they're called exercises, their purpose is to help you breathe correctly. When your breathing is correct, your sensitivity becomes normal, correcting not only distortion of the body but also any tendencies regarding appetite and emotions.

Here are some keys to the practice:

① Inhale deeply into your abdomen.

② Complete the movements on the exhalation, and try to push your stomach in.

③ Once you've completed a pose, do Corpse Pose for a few minutes or two to balance your breath.

These won't be effective if you distort your breathing or practice with force. Even though these seem like physical exercises, remember they're really about breathing.

It's like when you yawn or stretch. Nobody intends to yawn. And when you stretch, you're not thinking about the direction and angle of your arms and legs. But once it's done, you feel refreshed and good, and your breath becomes easier. You can't force that to happen even if you want to. If you try to accomplish it intentionally, it doesn't feel as good as when you do it naturally.

The postures should be practiced when the time is right, and for the right amount of time. Here's how to figure that out.

One rule is to practice the postures you're least good at the most often, and to practice on the more difficult side. Other rules are as follows:

1. *Stretch any areas that are contracted.* Your breath will be more complete and deep when your muscles are flexible enough to stretch and contract. Stretching the difficult side as you exhale will naturally help you breathe more deeply and take in more oxygen.

2. *Soften any parts of the body that are stiff.* When your muscles are stiff and inflexible, the blood doesn't circulate well, gets congested easily, and is usually cold. To soften an area, move, pound, rub, or twist it.

3. *Straighten the parts of your body that are twisted.* If your pelvis is crooked, you'll be more prone to falling, ankle sprains, and backache. If, while doing active pose #1 (page 120): internal organ correcting pose A), you have a hard time doing it on one side, it means that your body is crooked in the opposite direction.

4. *Strengthen any areas that are weak.* If the muscles on one side of your leg, arm abdomen, or back are stronger, the balance of your internal organs will be affected. Because we tend to use our stronger hand or foot in daily life, we end up training one side of our body more rigorously. Do the opposite on purpose, and strengthen the weaker or less used side.

5. *Stretch the shorter side and contract the longer side.* Compare the right and left sides of your arms and legs, and stretch the shorter one and contract the longer one. In exercise 2, for example, if you stretch your shorter leg while you lift your hip and twist it to both sides, you'll give your body what it needs.

6. *Loosen areas that are tight and tighten areas that are loose.* It's optimal to achieve a balance between tension (tightness) and relaxation (looseness). If the body is tight or loose, it's not stable. Try to get to the point where you can do everything with equal strength and ease, such as separating your legs and moving your arms to the front, back, left, and right.

7. *Balance your force.* A crooked posture causes imbalance in the elasticity of our muscles, and will transform the shape of the bones and internal organs. You may tend to carry heavy things with your stronger arm, which causes an imbalance. To counteract this, do push-ups with each arm, doing more repetitions with the weaker one, or train the weaker one with a dumbbell.

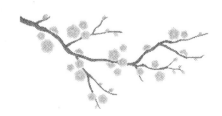

1. Internal organ correcting pose A

To enhance the flexibility of the internal organs and the spine and to make the internal organs more active.

①Lie on your back, knees bent, arms stretched to the side.

②As you exhale, bring both knees down to your right side; bring them back to center as you inhale. Repeat on the left.

③Continue this movement in harmony with your breath. Then repeat the exercise with both feet lifted off the floor, knees in toward your chest.

Doing this exercise with the feet slightly off the floor stimulates the stomach and liver. When the knees are brought to the chest, it stimulates the kidneys. This posture improves blood circulation in the area by repeatedly contracting and expanding the entire abdominal area.

2. Internal organ correcting pose B

To strengthen the spine and foster blood circulation in the lower abdomen, improving functioning.

①Lie on your back, fingers interlaced behind your neck, elbows open.

②Lift your hips as high as you can. As you exhale, twist your hips to the right. Come back to center as you inhale, then exhale and twist to the left.

③Repeat, opening the legs slightly wider each time.

Keeping the feet hip-width apart stimulates the upper spine and kidneys. As you open your legs, first the lower spine and then the intestines are stimulated.

1. Internal organ correcting pose A

2. Internal organ correcting pose B

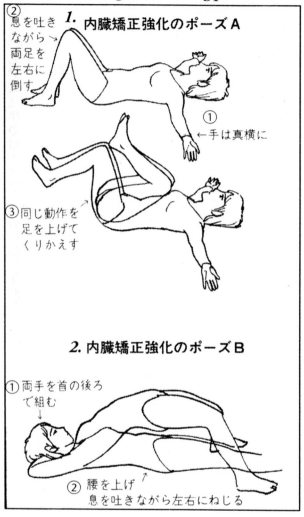

1. 内臓矯正強化のポーズ A

② 息を吐きながら両足を左右に倒す

① ←手は真横に

③ 同じ動作を足を上げてくりかえす

2. 内臓矯正強化のポーズ B

① 両手を首の後ろで組む
↓

② 腰を上げ
息を吐きながら左右にねじる

3. Internal organ correcting pose C

To strengthen the muscles in the sides and legs.

① Lie on your back and lift your legs perpendicular to the floor, feet pointed. Support your body with your arms at your sides. Take a deep breath, hold it, and concentrate on your tanden.

② As you breathe out forcefully, turn your legs to the right, feet together. Stop just before the legs touch the floor, and bring them back to the center as you inhale. Keep your left shoulder on the floor.

③ Repeat on the left. Continue. Doing both sides counts as one repetition.

4. Pelvis correcting pose A

To strengthen tanden.

① Sit on the floor between your bent legs (wariz position)

② With your arms straight in front of you, twist your wrists forcefully toward center. Lie back on the floor and take a deep breath.

③ Tuck in your chin and slowly lift your upper body as you exhale bit by bit.

④ Focus on tanden throughout the exercise.

⑤ Keeping your wrists twisted, exhale and bend forward. Touch the floor with your stomach and forehead.

⑥ Inhale and lift your upper body to the original position.

3. Internal organ correcting pose C

4. Pelvis correcting pose A

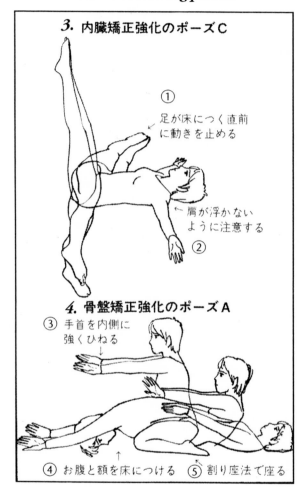

3. 内臓矯正強化のポーズC

① 足が床につく直前に動きを止める

← 肩が浮かないように注意する ②

4. 骨盤矯正強化のポーズA

③ 手首を内側に強くひねる

④ お腹と額を床につける　⑤ 割り座法で座る

5. *Pelvis correcting pose B*

To balance flexibility on both sides of the pelvis and make the bones flexible.

①Lie on your back, feet twisted inward, legs wide apart.

②Hold your arms straight up, wrists twisted inward and the backs of the hands touching.

③Lift your head as you inhale, and hold your breath. Focus on tanden.

④As you exhale slowly, stretch your arms forward, the backs of the hands still together. Lift the upper body halfway up, and hold your breath. Be careful not to strain your shoulders and don't bend your knees.

⑤With your force still in tanden, lift your upper body all the way up.

6. *Pelvis correcting pose C*

To make the pelvis flexible.

①Bend your right leg and place it over the groin of your left thigh. Stretch your left Achilles tendon and take a deep breath.

②Focus your mind on tanden and bend forward with your arms stretched in front as you exhale forcefully.

③Keep bending, with your right knee pressed against the floor, until your forehead touches your leg below your left knee.

④Grab your left toes with both hands and stretch your Achilles tendon, keeping your elbows on the floor.

⑤Hold your breath as long as possible in this posture.

⑥When you can't hold it anymore, relax and slowly raise your upper body as you inhale.

5. *Pelvis correcting pose B*

6. *Pelvis correcting pose C*

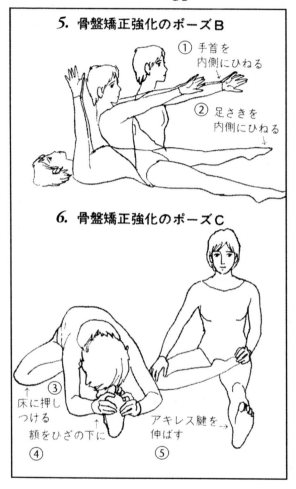

5. 骨盤矯正強化のポーズB

① 手首を内側にひねる

② 足さきを内側にひねる

6. 骨盤矯正強化のポーズC

③ 床に押しつける

④ 額をひざの下に

⑤ アキレス腱を伸ばす

7. Pelvis correcting pose D

To make the pelvis flexible.

① Lie on your back. Bend your left leg and pull the heel in close to the top of the inner thigh. Keep the right leg straight and slightly open. Be sure to keep your left knee on the floor.

② Interlace your fingers and, turning your hands palms facing out, stretch your arms up. Relax your shoulders.

③ Lift your head as you inhale, and hold your breath. Focus all your power in your tanden.

④ Lift your upper body halfway up as you exhale slightly, then hold your breath again.

⑤ Lift your upper body all the way up as you exhale forcefully.

8. Pelvis correcting pose E

To strengthen the inner thighs and enhance abdominal pressure.

① Lie on your back and bend your right leg below the knee to the side, as in Hero Pose (Virasana). Stretch both Achilles tendons.

② Grab your right ankle with your right hand, placing your left hand on your left lower abdomen.

③ Take a deep breath and slowly lift your upper body as you exhale little by little.

④ Push against the floor with your right knee, trying not to let your legs open.

⑤ Repeat with the left leg bent.

NOTE:

⑥ Stretch your Achilles tendon.

⑦ Place your left hand on your left lower abdomen.

7. *Pelvis correcting pose D*

8. *Pelvis correcting pose E*

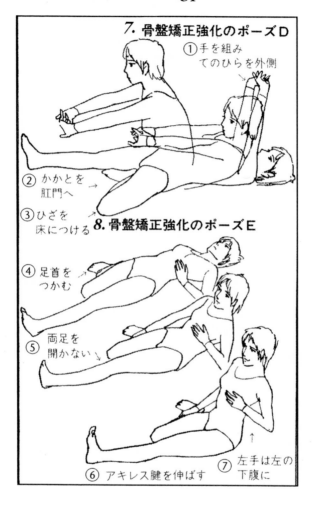

7. 骨盤矯正強化のポーズD

① 手を組み
てのひらを外側

② かかとを
肛門へ →

③ ひざを
床につける

8. 骨盤矯正強化のポーズE

④ 足首を
つかむ

⑤ 両足を
開かない ↓

⑥ アキレス腱を伸ばす

⑦ 左手は左の
下腹に ↑

9. Pelvis correcting pose F

To make the pelvis flexible.

①Lie on your back. Bend your left leg below the knee to the side, as in Hero Pose (Virasana) and grab your toes with your left hand.

②Keep your right leg straight and open, and your right arm straight at your side.

③Take a deep breath and hold it. Bring power to your tanden.

④Exhale forcefully and, keeping your left knee on the floor, lift the tip of your left foot.

⑤Continue exhaling. Once you've exhaled completely, drop your left foot on the floor.

⑥Repeat with the right foot.

10. Balance correcting pose A

To stimulate the upper backbone; to balance liver function (when turning to the left) and stomach and pancreas (when turning to the right); to treat back pain.

①Get into Cat Pose. Bring your elbows to your sides, and try to keep your chest on the floor.

②Inhale and hold, focusing on tanden.

③Sending power to your tanden, press against the floor with your right elbow and slowly turn your hip to the left as you exhale forcefully. Focus your attention on the muscles in the right side of the body.

④Keep turning until your left thigh is slightly above the floor, and continue exhaling. When you've exhaled completely, relax in the pose and hold your breath for a while.

⑤Inhale and come back to center.

⑥Repeat on the right.

9. Pelvis correcting pose F

10. Balance correcting pose A

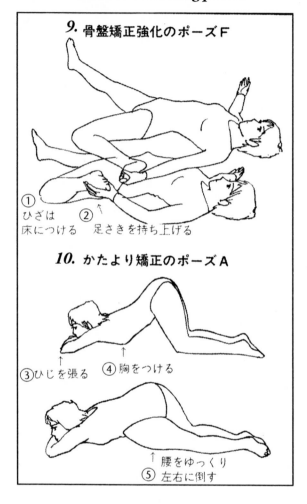

9. 骨盤矯正強化のポーズF

① ひざは
床につける　② ↑　足さきを持ち上げる

10. かたより矯正のポーズA

③ ひじを張る　④ ↑　胸をつける

↑ 腰をゆっくり
⑤ 左右に倒す

11. Balance correcting pose B

To solve atrophy of the right and left sides of the chest; to correct problems in the side and upper back muscles; to correct crookedness in the spine; to stimulate the lungs, liver, and especially the large intestines.

① Lie on your stomach with your forehead on the floor. Place your right hand on your neck and your left hand on your hip.

② Take a deep breath and hold it, lift your head and slowly arch your back, keeping your force in tanden.

③ Once you've arched your upper body as far as possible, hold it for a while.

④ Focus your attention on the left side of your hip and turn your upper body to the left as you exhale forcefully. Keep your right elbow up. Once you've turned and exhaled completely, relax in the position.

12. Balance correcting pose C

To correct blood circulation problems in the chest and dislocation of the internal organs.

① Lie on your back, knees bent 90 degrees and arms stretched straight to the side.

② Lift your hip as you inhale, and hold your breath, focusing on your tanden.

③ Turn your focus to your pelvis, lifting your hip higher as you exhale forcefully, and turn both knees to the right.

④ Lower your knees as far as possible without touching the floor. Hold the posture while you continue exhaling. Stretch your left arm, keep your right leg strong, and relax your left leg.

⑤ As you finish exhaling, relax in the posture.

11. Balance correcting pose B

12. Balance correcting pose C

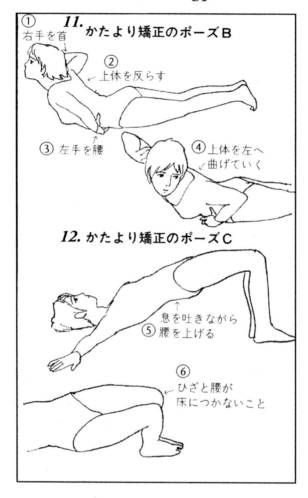

① 右手を首

11. かたより矯正のポーズB

② 上体を反らす

③ 左手を腰

④ 上体を左へ 曲げていく

12. かたより矯正のポーズC

⑤ 息を吐きながら 腰を上げる

⑥ ひざと腰が 床につかないこと

13. Balance correcting pose D

To correct the location of the pelvis and shoulder blades; to treat problems in the large intestines, eyes, ears, nose, hands and feet, as well as back pain.

① Beginning in seiza, slide your buttocks to the left and sit sideways.

② Interlace your fingers behind your neck, keeping your elbows parallel, and focus on your tanden.

③ Keeping your force in your tanden, focus on your left abdomen and bend your upper body to the right as you exhale forcefully.

④ Put all your weight on your right buttock and bend as far as you can. When you finish exhaling, relax in the posture. Return to center and repeat the bend on your left.

14. Balance correcting pose E

To contract the muscles in the legs and side of the abdomen; to correct hip problems and crookedness in the spine; to enhance the functioning of the internal organs and blood circulation.

① Kneel with your knees hip width apart. Take a deep breath and bring force to your tanden. Relax your arms.

② Push against the floor with your knees and exhale forcefully as you push your hips to the front and bend your upper body backward.

③ Grab your right ankle with your right hand and stretch and lift your left arm, drawing an arc. Then pull it down toward your head.

④ Continue exhaling. Push out your hips and try to bring your left hand closer to the floor.

⑤ As you finish exhaling, relax in the posture.

13. Balance correcting pose D

14. Balance correcting pose E

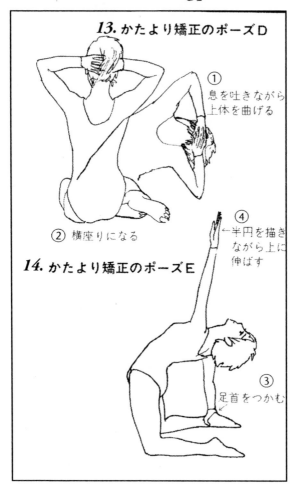

13. かたより矯正のポーズD

① 息を吐きながら
上体を曲げる

② 横座りになる

14. かたより矯正のポーズE

④ ←半円を描き
ながら上に
伸ばす

③ 足首をつかむ

15. Balance correcting pose F

To treat problems caused by a lowering of one side of the ribs or by differences in strength of the left and right hands.

① Get into push-up position with one hand in front of the other. If one shoulder is generally lower than the other, place that hand in front.

② Take a deep breath and bring force to your tanden. Slowly bend your elbows as you exhale forcefully.

③ When your body is slightly above the floor, hold your breath.

④ Continue exhaling and stretch your arms out to lift your body. Return to the original position as you finish exhaling. Repeat several times.

16. Balance correcting pose G

To correct crookedness caused by difference in strength between the left and right sides of the chest or abdominal muscles.

① If your left arm and leg are contracted: Get on your stomach, bend your right leg, and grab the bottom part of your lower leg with your right hand.

② Take a deep breath and focus on your tanden, collecting force into it.

③ Lift your right arm and leg, arching your body, as you exhale forcefully, and stretch your left arm and leg as much as you can. Try not to bend the left knee. Your attention is on your right hip.

④ When you've exhaled completely, relax in the posture.

⑤ If your right arm and leg are contracted: Complete the posture on the opposite side.

15. Balance correcting pose F

16. Balance correcting pose G

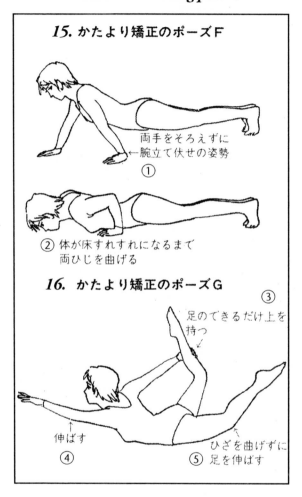

15. かたより矯正のポーズF

両手をそろえずに
←腕立て伏せの姿勢
①

② 体が床すれすれになるまで
両ひじを曲げる

16. かたより矯正のポーズG

③

足のできるだけ上を
持つ
↙

伸ばす
↑
④

ひざを曲げずに
⑤ 足を伸ばす

17. Forward/backward entrenched bend correcting pose A

To correct and to strengthen the abdominal muscles by enhancing their flexibility; to treat muscle tightness in the front thigh.

① Sit with your legs to the side, as in Hero Pose (Virasana). Bring your upper body down and lie on your back.

② Place your hands under your lower back, palms facing down.

③ Lift your hips, take a deep breath, and hold it. Gather force in your tanden and focus your attention on your pelvis.

④ As you exhale forcefully, lift your hips higher and try to move your hands toward your head. (Don't strain your hips when you lift them; instead, lift by stretching your knees and back muscles.)

⑤ Once you've exhaled completely, relax in the posture.

18. Forward/backward entrenched bend correcting pose B

To correct humpback and to strengthen the big toes and lower back and abdomen, which heals congestion in the lower abdomen.

① Lie on your back. Lift your arms perpendicular to the floor, fingers straight. Bend your legs and place your feet flat on the floor.

② As you take a deep breath, lift your head, hold your breath, and concentrate force into your tanden.

③ Strengthen your big toes and lift your upper body half way as you exhale slightly, then hold your breath again.

④ Focus on your abdomen.

⑤ Lift your upper body all the way up as you exhale completely.

⑥ Once you've exhale completely, relax in the posture.

17. *Forward/backward entrenched bend correcting pose A*

18. *Forward/backward entrenched bend correcting pose B*

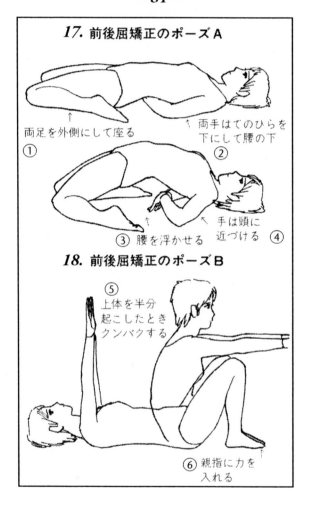

17. 前後屈矯正のポーズA

① 両足を外側にして座る

② 両手はてのひらを下にして腰の下

③ 腰を浮かせる

④ 手は頭に近づける

18. 前後屈矯正のポーズB

⑤ 上体を半分起こしたときクンバクする

⑥ 親指に力を入れる

19. Forward/backward entrenched bend correcting pose C

To stretch the chest muscle up and down and treat tightness in the leg and hip muscles.

① Lie on your stomach with your legs straight together and your hands on the floor next to your chest.

② Lift your head slightly as you take a deep breath and hold it, focusing your attention in your tanden.

③ With force in your tanden, lift your upper body as you exhale forcefully. At the same time, bend your knees and bring your toes toward your head. Straighten your arms, increase the force in your fingers, and push out your chin.

④ Focus on the place in your spine that is feeling the most pressure and hold your breath again.

⑤ As you continue exhaling, arch your back even farther. Once you've exhaled completely, relax in the posture.

20. Forward/backward entrenched bend correcting pose D

To treat postures such as humpback.

① Lie on your stomach, knees bent, and grab your feet with both hands. Keep your knees hip-width apart.

② Take a deep breath and hold it. With force in your tanden, focus your attention on the back of your head. Exhale forcefully as you increase the strength in your elbows and push down on your feet with your hands so that your heels touch the floor.

③ Once your heels are on the floor, continue exhaling, push your toes down to the floor, and lift your head and upper chest. Push out your chin as if you're trying to touch your back with the back of your head.

④ Once you've exhaled completely, relax in the posture.

19. *Forward/backward entrenched bend correcting pose C*

20. *Forward/backward entrenched bend correcting pose D*

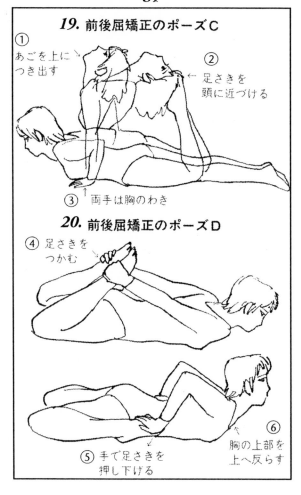

19. 前後屈矯正のポーズＣ

① あごを上に つき出す

② ← 足さきを 頭に近づける

③ ↑ 両手は胸のわき

20. 前後屈矯正のポーズＤ

④ 足さきを つかむ

⑤ 手で足さきを 押し下げる

⑥ 胸の上部を 上へ反らす

21. Forward/backward entrenched bend correcting pose E

To correct forward-bending postures caused by lack of strength in the stomach and chest muscles and contraction of the muscles in the front of the legs; to correct problems in the spine.

① Lie on your back. Bend your legs below the knees, as in Hero Pose (Virasana), heels by your hips, and grab your ankles.

② Take a deep breath and hold it, focusing your attention and force in your tanden.

③ Bring your focus to your pelvis and lift your hips and shoulders as you exhale forcefully, and touch the floor with the top of your head. Arch your body as if you're pushing your hips to the front.

④ Arch as far as possible. When you've exhaled completely, relax in the posture.

22. Crookedness correcting pose A

To correct crookedness throughout the body.

① Lie on your back with your right hand behind your head, elbow straight out, and your left hand straight at your side.

② Bend your right knee and lift it, keeping your left leg straight. Stretch your Achilles tendon.

③ Take a deep breath and hold it, focusing your mind on your tanden.

④ Lift your upper body half way and twist to the right as you exhale slightly. Stretch your left hand out in front of you, then bring the palm to the outside of the right knee. Push against the knee with your palm as you get up. Pull your right elbow back.

⑤ Exhale more forcefully and twist your upper body even farther to the right. Focus on the right side of your back.

⑥ Once you've finished twisting and have exhaled completely, relax and return to the original posture.

21. Forward/backward entrenched bend correcting pose E

22. Crookedness correcting pose A

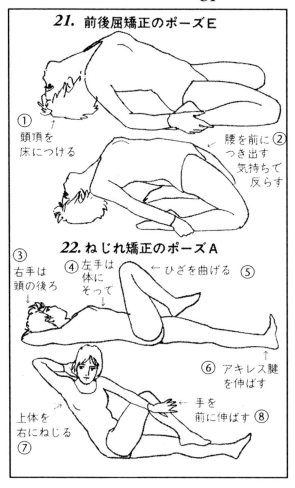

21. 前後屈矯正のポーズE

① 頭頂を床につける

② 腰を前につき出す気持ちで反らす

22. ねじれ矯正のポーズA

③ 右手は頭の後ろ

④ 左手は体にそって

⑤ ←ひざを曲げる

⑥ アキレス腱を伸ばす

⑦ 上体を右にねじる

⑧ ←手を前に伸ばす

23. Crookedness correcting pose B

To correct crookedness in the body caused by problems in lumbar vertabra #3.

① Sit on the floor with your left knee bent and your right leg straight in front of you. Place your hands shoulder-width apart behind you.

② Lift your hips, arch your chest, and take a deep breath. Hold it and lift your right leg slightly. As you exhale forcefully, bring the leg to the right. Focus on the area below your shoulder blades.

③ Relax your neck, stretch and strengthen your toes, and push out your chin. Try to keep your right leg as wide open as possible.

④ When you've exhaled completely, relax in the posture.

24. Crookedness correcting pose C

To correct crookedness in the spine and back muscles.

① Keeping your toes and knees straight, open your legs wide.

② Interlace your fingers behind your head, keeping your elbows on a straight line. Keep your spine straight.

③ Take a deep breath and focus your attention on your tanden.

④ Exhale slightly and twist your upper body to the left, focusing your attention on the right side of your back, and keeping force in your tanden.

⑤ Bend forward and to the left as if you're trying to touch your left leg with your upper body. Continue pushing your left elbow out forcefully, and keep your right leg stretched.

⑥ Bend as far as you can and touch your left knee with your right elbow. When you've exhaled completely, relax in the posture.

23. Crookedness correcting pose B

24. Crookedness correcting pose C

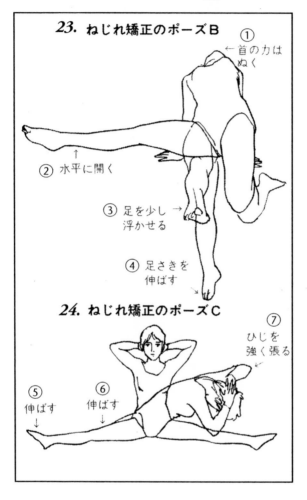

23. ねじれ矯正のポーズB

① ←首の力は ぬく

② 水平に開く

③ 足を少し 浮かせる

④ 足さきを 伸ばす

24. ねじれ矯正のポーズC

⑦ ひじを 強く張る

⑤ 伸ばす

⑥ 伸ばす

25. Crookedness correcting pose D

To correct crookedness in the body caused by a difference in strength between the abdominal and chest muscles.

① Lie on your stomach and stretch your arms out to the side, palms facing down, legs straight.

② Lift each leg up high, one at a time. Begin with your right leg: lift it high, take a deep breath, and hold it. Focus on your tanden.

③ As you exhale forcefully, lean your right leg toward the left side of your body, with your knee and toes straight. Focus on your right hip. Relax your left leg. Keep your chin and right shoulder on the floor and don't move your neck.

④ Try to lean your right leg as far toward the left side of your body as possible. When you've exhaled completely, relax in the posture and rest while breathing. Repeat on whichever side was more difficult.

26. Crookedness correcting pose E

To correct torsion and to adjust any differences in strength between the left and right sides and upper and lower parts of the lateral muscles and the muscles around the ribcage and shoulder blades.

① Beginning in Cat Pose (p.29), choose the leg that's more difficult to lift and lift it as high as possible.

② Take a deep breath and hold it. Concentrate your focus on your tanden and gather strength into it.

③ As you exhale forcefully, straighten the toes of the foot that's lifted and turn the foot toward the opposite side (in other words, if your left leg is lifted, turn it to the right). As you do so, focus on the flank of the lifted leg.

④ Continue exhaling. When you can't hold any longer, relax in the posture.

25. *Crookedness correcting pose D*

26. *Crookedness correcting pose E*

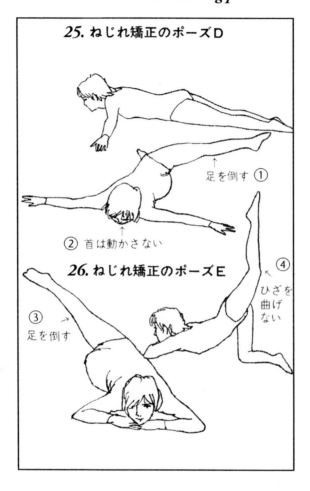

25. ねじれ矯正のポーズD

足を倒す ①

② 首は動かさない

26. ねじれ矯正のポーズE

④
ひざを曲げない

③
足を倒す

27. Crookedness correcting pose F

To correct crookedness caused by vertical movements of the pelvis and by difference in muscle strength in the left and right hips.

① Sit in seiza. Shift your weight to your left buttock and lay your feet on the floor outside of your right hip, with your left ankle resting in the left arch. Try to repeat by shifting to the right side. Choose the side that's more difficult. (For the purposes of this example, we'll start with the left side.)

② Keep your spine straight and interlace your fingers behind your head, elbows forming a straight line parallel to the floor.

③ Take a deep breath and hold it, focusing on your tanden.

④ Focus your attention on your right abdomen and turn your upper body as you exhale forcefully, extending your right knee as though you were pushing it forward as far as you can.

⑤ Twist as far as you can. When you've exhaled completely, relax in the posture.

⑥ Inhale slowly and come back to center.

⑦ Repeat on the right.

28. Elevated-center-of-gravity correcting pose A

To correct a condition in which the body's center moves upward due to fatigue and other conditions in the head, causing cramping in the Achilles tendons. (Your center of gravity should be found in your tanden; however, when you are tired, angry, or upset, the center often moves up toward your head, neck, and shoulder areas); to tighten the scalp and improve blood circulation in the head.

① Lie on your back and interlace your fingers behind your head.

② Take a deep breath and hold it. Focus your mind on your tanden.

③ Exhale forcefully as you strengthen your elbows and stretch your Achilles tendons, while pushing against the floor with your elbows. Tuck in your chin and open your chest. Push your head up with your hands, keeping your neck straight.

④ Concentrate your focus on the back of your head as you continue exhaling. Relax as you exhale completely.

27. *Crookedness correcting pose F*

28. *Elevated-center-of-gravity correcting pose A*

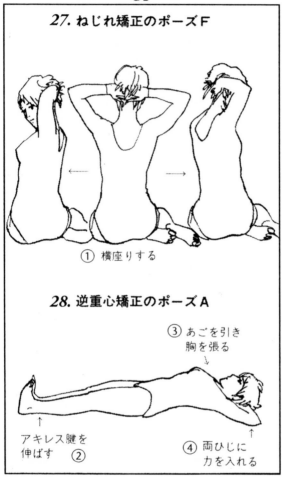

27. ねじれ矯正のポーズF

① 横座りする

28. 逆重心矯正のポーズA

③ あごを引き
胸を張る

アキレス腱を
伸ばす ②

④ 両ひじに
力を入れる

29. Elevated-center-of-gravity correcting pose B

To correct a condition in which the body's center moves upward due to stiffness in the neck and shoulders; to loosen the neck and shoulders and improve blood circulation in the head.

① Lie on your back with your elbows at right angles and make fists with your hands next to your hips.

② Take a deep breath and hold it. Concentrate your focus on your tanden to strengthen it.

③ As you exhale forcefully, strengthen your elbows, stretch your Achilles tendons, and tuck in your chin. Push against the floor with your elbows and stick out your chest. Slide your elbows along the floor toward your head.

④ Concentrate your focus on the base of your neck.

⑤ Continue exhaling as you keep moving your elbows toward your head. Relax as you exhale completely.

30. Elevated-center-of-gravity correcting pose C

To release excess tension in the chest and to correct the location of the body's center by eliminating stiffness.

① Lie on your back with your elbows bent at right angles. Make fists with your hands and place them by your head.

② Take a deep breath and hold it. Concentrate your attention on your tanden.

③ Strengthen your hands and elbows to push against the floor. As you exhale forcefully, lift and stick out your chest as if you're trying to bring your shoulder blades together. Tuck in your chin and stretch your Achilles tendons.

④ Focus on your shoulder blades.

⑤ Continue exhaling and hold as long as you can. When you've exhaled completely, relax in the posture.

29. Elevated-center-of-gravity correcting pose B

30. Elevated-center-of-gravity correcting pose C

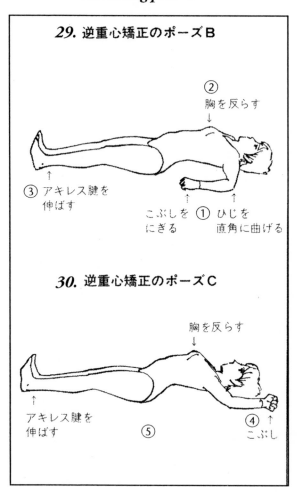

29. 逆重心矯正のポーズ**B**

② 胸を反らす

③ アキレス腱を
伸ばす

こぶしを ① ひじを
にぎる 直角に曲げる

30. 逆重心矯正のポーズ**C**

胸を反らす

アキレス腱を
伸ばす
⑤

④ こぶし

31. Elevated-center-of-gravity correcting pose D

A stronger version of elevated-center-of-gravity correcting pose A. To strengthen the abdomen and legs and to enhance the ability of the pelvis to open and close flexibly.

① Lie on your back and interlace your fingers behind your neck. Keep your legs straight and your toes together, with your heels as wide apart as possible.

② Take a deep breath and hold it. Tuck in your chin as you exhale. Stretch your elbows out to the side. Stretch the lower back of your head with both your hands behind it as you stretch your Achilles tendons, keeping your feet slightly off the floor.

③ Focus on the back of your head.

④ Continue exhaling in the posture. When you've exhaled completely, relax.

32. Elevated-center-of-gravity correcting pose E

A stronger version of elevated-center-of-gravity correcting pose C. To lift the feet in order to lower a center that's too high; to stimulate the upper right-hand area of the body by moving both feet to the right.

① As in pose C, bend your elbows at right angles, keeping your fists by your head.

② Inhale and hold. Lift your feet slightly off the floor.

③ Gather force in your tanden and push out your chest as you push against the floor with your hands and elbows. Focus on the upper-right hand portion of your chest.

④ As you exhale, stretch your Achilles tendons and stick out your chest even farther and bring both legs to the left.

⑤ Relax as you exhale completely.

31. Elevated-center-of-gravity correcting pose D

32. Elevated-center-of-gravity correcting pose E

31. 逆重心矯正のポーズD

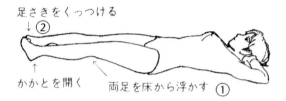

足さきをくっつける
②

かかとを開く　　両足を床から浮かす　①

32. 逆重心矯正のポーズE

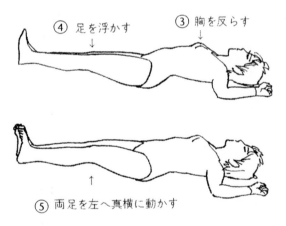

④ 足を浮かす　　③ 胸を反らす

⑤ 両足を左へ真横に動かす

33. Elevated-center-of-gravity correcting pose F:

To correct a condition in which the center is too high because the hips lack strength and the chest and upper back are congested.

①Lie on your stomach, bend your elbows, and keep the back of your hands on the floor.

②Keeping your elbows on the floor, move them toward your head as you inhale. Once the back of your hands touch your armpits, hold your breath. Focus on your tanden and strengthen it.

③Bring your attention to your shoulder blade. As you exhale forcefully, push your elbows toward your head and lift your legs as if you're pushing up your pelvis.

④Exhale completely and relax your elbows, staying in the posture.

34. Hip and abdomen strengthening pose A:

A variation on a push-up. To enhance the ability of the pelvis to open and close; to activate the nerves, hormones, and internal organs; to improve elimination.

①Get on all fours. Open your legs wide and place your hands in front of you, slightly more than shoulder-width apart.

②As you take a deep breath, stick your buttocks out in back and pull your chin to your chest.

③Keeping your heels on the floor, push your buttocks back and bring your face closer to the floor. Hold your breath.

④Exhale forcefully and slowly push your upper body forward, jutting out your chin.

⑤When your upper body is pushed as far forward as possible, drop your hips dramatically, straighten your elbows, and arch your entire body as you exhale completely. If possible, try to repeat this exercise thirty times in rapid succession without pausing.

33. *Elevated-center-of-gravity correcting pose F*

34. *Hip and abdomen strengthening pose A*

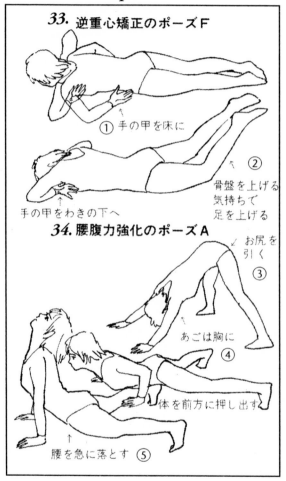

33. 逆重心矯正のポーズF

① 手の甲を床に

② 骨盤を上げる 気持ちで 足を上げる

手の甲をわきの下へ

34. 腰腹力強化のポーズA

お尻を 引く

③

あごは胸に

④

体を前方に押し出す

腰を急に落とす ⑤

35. Hip and abdomen strengthening pose B

To enhance the functioning of the intestines by tightly twisting the wrists, ankles, and hips.

① Place your feet wide apart with your hands on the floor, shoulder-width apart, elbows straight. Support your lower body with your toes.

② Keep your arms straight up from the floor and drop your hips low.

③ Twist your upper body and head to the left and try to look at your left heel. Twist both feet left so that both heels lean left.

④ Twist to the other side in the same manner. Repeat the movement as rapidly as possible.

⑤ Exhale when you twist and inhale when you come back to center.

⑥ Focus your attention on the heel that you're looking at.

36. Hip and abdomen strengthening pose C

To strengthen the hips and abdomen.

① Lie on your stomach with your elbows on the floor.

② Lift your body using only the toes and elbows. Keep your body parallel to the floor.

③ Inhale, and as you exhale, shift your body to the front and back.

④ Exhale as you shake your hips right and left.

⑤ As you complete these movements, focus on and keep strength in your tanden.

⑥ Exhale as you move your body back and forth and left and right, and inhale as you come back to center.

35. Hip and abdomen strengthening pose B

36. Hip and abdomen strengthening pose C

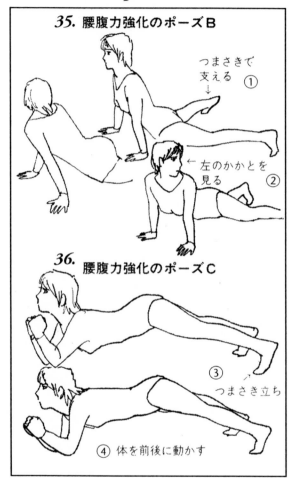

35. 腰腹力強化のポーズＢ

つまさきで
支える
↓
①

← 左のかかとを
見る
②

36. 腰腹力強化のポーズＣ

③
つまさき立ち

④ 体を前後に動かす

3. HAVE A FLEXIBLE AND STRONG KOKORO (HEART/MIND)

Humans are animals that reflect on what they've done. That's why we notice that something is wrong with our mind when we fail or make mistakes. But it's difficult to change our mind to make it the way we'd like it to be.

When you're studying for exams and need to concentrate, for example, you instead become restless and anxious. You get nervous before the exam. Or you get nervous when you meet new people, and are hesitant to express your thoughts the way you'd like to.

These things happen because failures and mistakes we've made in the past build up, and also because of bad habits. When you have two different thoughts in your mind, the stronger one always wins out at the end. Whatever is more familiar to you—whatever you've repeated and practiced—is stronger.

When a bad habit of your mind wins, it becomes a problem. To prevent this from happening, you must first change the physical aspects. You train your body through the experiences of the physical training I've introduced. In other words, you train your mind with physical training during living and working. You purify, strengthen, and alter your mind through everything you do. Learning everything from our teacher – nature – is a way of life. The techniques I've introduced are a way to use the body to strengthen the mind.

Here, I'd like to discuss some more practical techniques to strengthen the mind – to create a stable mind when you need to be calm and a flexible mind when you need to be active.

Techniques to balance the mind by moving the body

If you feel that your mind isn't calm, try the following movements.

To calm yourself down. For when you get nervous easily at exams or interviews, and can't do your best; when you blush or find it difficult to speak when you meet people.

In situations like these, your energy is in your shoulders, neck, and hands, and not in your legs or hips.

A. Try to move the energy to your lower abdomen by jumping or doing shiko like a sumo wrestler.

B. Bring force into your legs, crouch down, stick out your chest, and take a deep breath to calm down.

To feel more active. For when you have to work, but you don't feel like doing anything; when you get up in the morning and don't feel like going to school.

You don't have energy because your hip is stiff, your neck lacks strength, and your chin is jutting out.

B. As you exhale forcefully, expand your chest, pull in your chin, and move your arms as if you're punching the space in front of you with your fists.

C. Stand on tiptoe and take a deep breath, filling your chest. Pull your hands in back of you and quickly swing them to the front. Hold your breath for a moment and then crouch down and exhale at once.

To control your desires. For when you can't manage chores, study, or work because you have a strong sex drive or appetite.

Your energy is in your neck and shoulders, and your blood is in your head because you're humpbacked.

A. The Headstand Pose is effective.

B. Lift your shoulders up and down and rotate your neck. Then, placing your hands on your hips and arching your back, take some deep breath to open the chest muscles, pelvis, and knees.

To clear your mind. For when you lack new ideas; when your memory is vague and you can't concentrate.

When you sit in a chair for a long time, your Achilles tendons get cramped.

A. Step forward with one leg, hands on your hips. As you exhale, stretch your Achilles tendon. Come back to center as you inhale, and step forward with the other leg.

B. Stand up. Exhale as you twist your arms toward center. Inhale as you twist your arms away from center. Repeat about five times.

This is like first-aid for a temporary change in attitude. To strengthen your mind, you need to look deep inside it and know its system.

A strong mind is created through five qualities: 1) flexibility, 2) stability, 3) enlightenment, 4) application ability, and 5) positive attitude. Let's look at each of these.

Making your mind flexible

A flexible, soft mind is a mind that can get along with anyone and enjoy any situation.

When I was younger, I thought having a strong mind meant having the capacity to exert yourself. So I endured anything by clenching my teeth, and I also tried hard to push my ideas forward. But as I studied yoga, I came to understand what real strength is about. Strength of mind can be attained only when your mind is soft and relaxed and you have a joyful life.

In Japan, we have a saying: "A willow will never break because of heavy snow" ("It's better to bend than to break"). The strongest tree is not the one that's sturdy and doesn't bend with the wind, but rather a willow, which yields to the wind. Sturdy trees break in a storm or heavy snow, but willows remain the same after a disaster, even if they were about to fall in the middle of it.

People complain that they're troubled, that they dislike something, or that they're stuck. But when willows' branches are bent, they don't feel they can't take it anymore. They know how to dodge hardships skillfully. The way that willows live suits the law of nature, and it's applicable to us humans.

So how can we attain flexibility and softness of mind? Flexibility is, to use another term, expansiveness of mind. The mind is more flexible when there's a larger gap between the ability to contract and stretch, or between the forgiving mind and the unforgiving mind, or between hate and love. So when you don't like something, just dislike it thoroughly. If you spend your time thinking about why you don't like it or how you can grow to like it, the gap narrows more and more. Eventually, because humans can't stick with a feeling for a long time, you'll get tired of this feeling of dislike. That's the time to start thinking of a way to like something you dislike.

Not wanting to work or study is natural. You'd be lying if you said you totally enjoyed a difficult job or boring study. It's impossible to feel that way. If something is unpleasant, try to find a way to do it that's fun even though you don't like it. If you practice giving opposite stimulation to your mind or your body simultaneously, it will become flexible.

But doing only what you like is an unbalanced way of thinking. If you focus your energy to one side, your mind will be unbalanced as well. You need to be well balanced. This will be more fruitful if the gap between studying and playing, or scolding and praising, is large.

The way to balance your mind is to practice having simultaneously contradictory minds at all times.

Stabilizing your mind

In today's society, many people get upset over little things. These people are mentally unstable and have weak minds. If any problem surpasses their ability, they get anxious and nervous, and start complaining about others.

The human mind is stable in the face of what's known but unstable when facing the unknown. Delusion, illusion, misunderstanding, anxiety, and worry don't come from what's known.

But since humans are animals that think, we can't leave things unknown. Even if we don't really know something, we subconsciously want to believe we understand it. As a result, we often believe what other people say without judging. We feel relieved when we sympathize with someone and believe that we understand them. But that definitely won't stabilize the mind. Rather, it's like joining a fanatical religious organization. When you look back, you may wonder why you threw yourself into such a thing, but while you're in it, you don't realize how abnormal your mind is.

So in order to stabilize your mind, you have to train yourself to distinguish between what's known to you and what's unknown. For example, someone who is fasting for the first time might panic, believing that they'll die from not eating. But someone who has experienced fasting for a week or so can be calm while fasting for half a month.

Modern people amass a lot of information and are excessively protective of their materially abundant lifestyle, but what they really know is very little. They get nervous and lose themselves over little things. There are many suicide cases with unknown cause, but these people didn't choose to die after pondering their lives deeply or experiencing a deep sorrow. They just didn't know what to do, got nervous because nobody told them what to do, and suddenly killed themselves. It's difficult in such a case for the people around them to sense or expect the death that's coming.

The known world is a world of philosophy or science, and the unknown world is a world of religion. What modern men need is religion.

Things can only be the way they are. There are things you can't understand even if you try hard. The world of religion is where you let yourself flow with the law of nature, be empty, and get into a state of "letting be." To do this, you need to ponder the way you live and grasp your identity. You need to understand clearly what you should make yourself do in a given situation.

In order to feel comfortable in a chair, for example, the chair has to be right for you. In the same manner, it's natural that your way of thinking is different from others'. It's also important to find something that you truly admire, trust, and fall for. That's the only way to achieve freedom and growth. Copying someone is like being a slave.

Being enlightened

The important thing is to have your own thoughts. At the same time, those thoughts must be truthful enough to convince others.

When someone who's inexperienced makes a claim, they may appear to have strong intentions, but in fact they're just being persistent about what little knowledge they do have. They're not really expressing their truth or the world's truth. They're more concerned about their convenience or profit.

A truth is something convincing to others at a fundamental level despite small differences in opinion. It's not really about expressing your opinions.

Can you tell the difference in the following two sentences?

Humans sing songs.

Songs are sung by humans.

The former is centered on humans, and the latter on songs.

When you express your opinion, you center it on the truth. In other words, when you speak you should focus on the truth and not your ideas.

The astronomer Galileo Galilei was accused of claiming a heretical theory – that the earth was spinning. But this wasn't about his loss or gain, it was about truth.

It's wrong for someone to always talk about themselves as "I am…" or "But I am…" Nobody has ever talked me down, because I never say what I don't know. I never say what I haven't substantiated, understood, or experienced.

So how do we attain enlightenment? Enlightenment is about your mind becoming one with the truth. It's understanding the truth of things and incorporating that truth into your way of thinking and living. I am the only Masahiro Oki on this planet, so I have to find my way of living on my own. If you don't know or if you have no thoughts on how to manage certain matters, you can't grow as a human. You're lost.

Our society should be a gathering place of the enlightened. If a sheep runs off into a cliff, other sheep follow. But this should never happen in human society. We shouldn't be slaves to someone else's opinions.

Enhancing your application ability

Application ability is the power to turn your enemies into friends. Before you make negative statements like "That's not good," or "That's bad and harmful," think a way to help or uplift your enemies. You can't help being nervous as long as you think they're your enemies. When you're negative and passive like that, your mind can't be stable or strong. Love till the end, no matter how many times they betray you. If you get angry, you'll lose.

Application ability is love. Be friendly with people you don't like. Be grateful even when you get sick. Think of a way to like people, or to make the most of disease. It's also about praying.

A strong and flexible mind is created when you try, even though you don't like something.

What happens in the world and in the universe isn't caused by you. The only thing you can do, if anything, is to create a "condition" for what you expect to come true. The phenomenon happening in the world is happening regardless of your intention. Whatever happens is necessary in order to balance nature; nothing unnecessary happens. It rains because it's necessary; landslides occur because they're necessary. All humans can do is to make what's happening in the world useful and valuable – to apply everything toward the better. That's what religion is about.

Humans are said to be "beings," meaning that we use our life to enhance its value for ourselves and others. If we don't do anything, we are just survivors, like other animals, which live just to exist.

To find value in everything and to feel grateful is the beginning of religion or spiritual culture. Materialistic culture is great, but if we don't have a spiritual culture with which to appreciate it, our human society will be chaotic and fallen.

There is nothing more powerful than love (in other words, application ability), because it allows us to make the most of ourselves and others.

We can't live only for ourselves. We can't die without realizing the "love" hidden within us and applying it. We live by creating joy for ourselves and others.

Having a mind that affirms everything

Everything has good and bad sides. There's a good and bad side to being alone or being in a group, to city and country, to cold and heat. Everything has good and bad sides.

Focus on the good side and affirm everything. If you focus on the down side of a person, or of yourself, and are negative, you can't grow. The way we evaluate things is one-sided, so if you change your point of view, it can be positive. A quiet person isn't just quiet – they're someone who doesn't talk nonsense.

Having a positive mind is about accepting reality just as it is and having a mind of worship. If it rains, just be thankful. And then make use of it.

When you educate your children, you shouldn't say "it's bad" or "it's dangerous" too much. You should intentionally let your children experience difficulties so that they learn to accept the fact that there are stormy days and sunny days. Otherwise they won't grow strong.

So how do we maintain a positive mind? By living the way you are without pretending or wearing a mask. When I'm invited somewhere, I eat everything that's served. You should eat what someone cooks for you with love. I usually eat a little of what suits me, but I would never say, "I'm a vegetarian and eat brown rice" when I'm invited to a meal. Sometimes my body gets upset after I eat something that doesn't agree with me, but that's the way it is.

A really strong mind is wide, soft, peaceful, forgiving, and joyful. Yoga is a teaching that turns us into a good person with a deep and expansive mind rather than a narrow one. That's the principle of human mind. Every religion, ethic, and lesson should contain this. But to strengthen your mind, you need to better yourself by thinking with your head and applying this principle rather than listening to what other people tell you.

The purpose of yoga is to help you solve issues of your mind and body on your own. That's why we discuss just the general principles of mind and body.

Chapter 4

Capability of Mind and Body

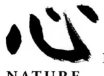

1. HAVE THE ABILITY TO FEEL NATURE

Modern men can only "feel" nature

The meditation practice that I'm about to discuss is the most important practice in yoga.

The postures, breathing techniques, and diet I've discussed are really preparation for meditation. They're *hatha* yoga, a practice that stabilizes the body and mind and corrects problems. Once your body and mind have been balanced and purified, you go on to *raja* yoga, a meditation practice. *Raja* yoga focuses primarily on the heart/mind. I'll explain these further.

It's easier to understand if you categorize the mind. Categorized into two parts, the mind is made up of "consciousness" and "unconsciousness." We could also add "subconscious awareness" and "universal consciousness"; in other words, *Shinshin-Betsubetsuno-Kokoro:* the mind/heart where it is separated from one's corporeity (a state in which there's knowledge only in the brain) and *Shinshin-Ittaino-Kokoro:* the mind/heart where it is one with one's corporeity, (a state in which the body incorporates the knowledge and makes it its own). It can also be categorized into *Sentenshin:* innate mind/heart (an innate instinct, like a baby drinking mother's milk) and *Kotenshin:* acquired mind/heart (something learned through training).

But the easiest way is to categorize it is by the action of the mind:

Kanjiru: to be aware, to sense
Omou: to believe
Kangaeru: to think

After you "think" thoroughly, it becomes "belief," and then the strong "belief" becomes "awareness."

The most important aspect to human life is "ways to be aware," but unfortunately modern humans must be trained to feel nature, or the universe, moment by moment, in other words, to be aware of or believe in nature or the universe instantaneously. We may think we feel it, but it's usually filtered through one's experiences or knowledge, which is different from really feeling it.

Yogic meditation is a training that enables us to think and feel expansively and deeply, and to look at things correctly.

You get sick because you don't feel

The ability to be aware is necessary in order to protect your own life. If you don't "feel good" or "become aware of goodness" toward things you need and "feel good" or "become aware of goodness" toward things you don't need, your mind/heart and body will react unnaturally and possibly betray you. If this ability is weak, you can't distinguish diseases or problems. If your feeling ability is strong, you have the intuition to discern things like "this is poisonous" or "I shouldn't do this." For example, if you continue to eat what you don't need, your body will create blood that's inappropriate for you. Then the nerves, muscles, and bones fed by this blood will become abnormal.

If you're trained solely to think like other people in today's society, your ability to feel will decay and your lifestyle will be wrong for you.

When we discover that we have a disease, we're too dependent on diagnosis, tests, and computers – in other words, intelligence. Our ability to feel is completely ignored. Diseases are symptoms that are expressed when our body senses problems and tries to eliminate them. So if we listen to our body, we'll know what treatment to use.

No matter how evolved we are, this ability to feel still functions as the basis of our life. Even though you can't see it, it's hidden deep within. It's our "sixth sense," a "hunch," or a "bad feeling."

Animals, by contrast, live only by feeling. They know well what they need, even though they're not taught what it is. Plants, for example, spread their roots and branches in an appropriate direction, and don't do anything that's not necessary. Anything that's unnecessary dies and falls off naturally. When there's too much snow on their branches and they're in danger of breaking, trees bend slowly to drop the snow. They seem to understand completely how to protect themselves.

Animals live very logically as well, without wasting anything, despite their lack of training. Elephants go to a special, unknown place to die because they have the ability to sense their own death. Humans are children born from nature, and we shouldn't forget to live according to nature's law. If we live using our ability to feel, we can be more true to our own lives.

Let's brush up on our "ability to feel" with the meditation practice that follows.

When you think, you're left with nothing but worries

Humans are said to be thinking animals. Humans became what they are because they had the ability to think and to learn. Therefore, we need to enhance our ability to think even further.

When we look at the history of the world, it's only recently that humans began to value thoughts over feelings. In ancient times and in the Middle Ages, the ability to feel was still present in the form of magic and mythology. While these had the power to guide humans, at the same time they contained aspects that could be considered illogical.

In our modern era, this aspect of human potential has been completely discarded because of the knowledge made up solely of "thoughts," called "science." Therefore, modern man lives by scientific rationality alone. All we think about is what to do or what not to do, and when something unknown happens, all we do is struggle and worry. At the very least, we should understand that thinking has its limits. We think based on our experiences, or what we've learned, so our thoughts are limited by our environment, our field of work, and other similar factors. So when we think without understanding, we can only act blindly. Therefore, we can have no idea whether we will succeed or fail, stay healthy or get sick.

Having a mind that's connected to the universe

Meditation is practiced to correct and enhance our way of feeling and thinking. In the practice, we teach to have no mind, but the first step is to have one mind (*Dharana*).

One mind means concentrating your mind strictly on one matter. When you look, focus only on looking. If you totally commit yourself to listening, walking, or thinking, your ability to feel will begin to cooperate. If you continue having one mind in this way, you'll come to have no mind.

If your mind is split, your ability to feel won't work. That's why you should be silent when you're troubled, instead of panicking. If you mind is quiet, you'll know what to do naturally.

When I was training in India, I was made to climb a mountain in the middle of the night and was left there alone without a guide. Even if it had been daylight, I wouldn't have known my way back. After some thought, I decided to give up and accept it as a training. And I meditated. Afterward, I knew which way to go naturally. My body must have remembered, even though my mind forgot. I walked for a while, and meditated whenever I was lost. As I kept at it, the wisdom of how to get back began to emerge.

Most people think wisdom is the ability to think, but it's not. Wisdom is feeling. But today, humans can only think. So we think and think. We need to stop thinking and quiet our minds. When you do this, the world you become aware of, the world you believe, and the world you think harmonize perfectly. You reach a state where your mind is in total unity. In yoga, this is called wisdom and in Buddhism, it's called Prajna, meaning pure and unqualified knowledge, or enlightenment. It's a mind that's in connection with the universe, nature, and god.

Meditation improves memory and uncovers telepathic ability

You can't deepen your understanding just by reading a lot of books or continuing to think. You'll just get confused. Take a break and meditate. Good thoughts usually come when you relax after working hard.

One way to improve your memory is to relax and quiet your mind after studying. After you've studied or memorized something, meditate about fifteen minutes before you go on to the next thing. If you try to learn something new right away, what you learned previously won't have enough time to sink into your head.

The same is true when you want to cultivate your ki power. Ki power isn't the power to think, but rather the energy within. Before you tell yourself to motivate, quiet your mind and make yourself feel good, and wait until your power naturally springs forward.

We often make mistakes in our sense of feeling when we keep humans at the center of our work or artistic activities. Keep the object at the center and have it teach you what to do. When you carve wood, ask the tree how it wants you to carve, or ask the plane how it wants you to use it. It's the same when you play the piano or release an arrow.

The key to doing better is to feel the object. To put it another way, listening to and feeling an object is seeing with your mind's eye. This mind's eye is also called the "third eye."

If your feeling ability improves, it becomes second sight, or telepathy. In the past, this was considered the "voice of god," and holy men and prophets practiced meditation deep in the mountains or desert to improve their intuition. When you hear the voice of god, it feels like it's coming from outside – but it really comes from within you. That may be why it's called divine revelation or affirmation.

When meditation practice has improved your ability to feel, you will, for example, know clearly what you need to eat right now. You'll know what yoga postures to take, how to stand or sit, and how to walk.

You already possess the basis of this. Everyone feels bad somehow after they've had bad thoughts or committed bad acts. You must have had an experience where something felt wrong and, looking back, you discovered there was a reason you felt that way.

If you improve your ability to physically sense when you feel bad, you can detect diseases before they get serious.

Practice using playful breaths

Every child has the ability to feel. This ability is lost when we grow up because the way we raise and educate children is incomplete.

Education today only trains us to improve our intelligence, and neglects the improvement of feeling. The study of art is supposed to train us to feel, but it's very brief and only teaches us the practice of following patterns. When students draw, they merely think of drawing beautifully like the examples they're given. It doesn't do anything. In true painting, you express how you feel through color and form. Dance and music are the same. Art is an expression of your joy or sadness through your body and music, without thought.

Play is the key to doing something well without using your mind. In play, there's no planning, or profit, or loss. You just do things to have fun, without worrying about whether you'll be praised or criticized, or whether or not you'll make money.

When you play, your breath is deep, long, and balanced. While this is one of the goals of yoga practice, it's also the key to doing anything.

When you're concerned about winning or losing, you become stressed and get sick when you're too exhausted. Study and work should be play. I'm active throughout the year, but I don't complain that "It's too much" or "I'm tired," because I'm really just playing.

Anyone can attain this kind of mindset by practicing meditation because it teaches you to attain a mind of detachment.

Principles of Shu (mimicry), Ha (breaking away), Ri (detachment, empty self, and rediscovery through connection with the universe)

Let's consider what it means to study yoga.

You begin studying something or learning an art by copying what other people feel, do, and think. But if all you do is copy, it never become yours – so you should consider copying a "priming water" that helps you create your own creation.

The principle to making your creation your own is composed of Shu, Ha, and Ri.

Shu means to copy a good teacher completely so that you can do the same thing. Ha means that, because something is borrowed from someone else, you refuse it and create your own. Ri means that if you meditate after every thought, you'll come up with a good idea. Likewise, if you let go of other people's thoughts as well as your own, within your emptiness you cultivate feeling, doing, and thinking that is connected to the universe. That is the principle of learning.

If you feel that something is "good," you should try to copy it. This also means to offer prayer or express your gratitude. It creates a suitable configuration within you. Then discard everything within that configuration that's borrowed, for now. When you stay away from what you've borrowed, you can create things that fit perfectly inside the configuration within you.

Becoming healthy through yoga postures is like that. Copy the right postures, then find your own stability on your own.

However, it is possible for you to have a bad teacher in the beginning of your studies, or your lack of understanding could cause you to develop a bad habit. If that happens, there's a way to change yourself: Dan, Sha, and Ri. If you have a bad habit, you must practice Dan (stop or give it up completely before it becomes permanent), and then practice Sha (discard or throw it out somewhere inaccessible), and then Ri (make it alien to you, something that is totally remote or has nothing to do with you). In yoga, for example, if you had a bad habit regarding preferences or amounts in terms of food consumption, you would practice Dan-Jiki, (Dan: stop or give up; Jiki: eating); i.e. fast, to allow your body to come up with new and different requirements. Dan also implies "eradicating the evil."

The ability to feel is buried within us, waiting to be unearthed

In the previous three steps of hatha yoga, we have done things to encourage natural breathing, because deep, long, and balanced breathing promotes our ability to feel.

In the fourth step, Pratyahara, we learn to exercise autogenous training in order to make this correct body and mind that we've learned completely our own.

In the fifth step, Dharana, we begin real meditation practice in order to train ourselves to focus our mind and harmonize our feeling and thinking.

In the sixth step, Dhyana, we empty our body and enhance it, and in the seventh step, bhakti, we empty our mind in order to enhance our spirituality.

In the eighth step, Samadhi, we try to attain the ability to feel completely. This step trains us to be Jitai-Ichinyo, meaning "others and (my)self are as one"—the philosophy that teaches that all lives are connected, no single life is isolated, and we are all deeply linked, in which other people's minds become like ours.

In the ninth step, Buddhi, we develop higher spirituality in its totality within our body and mind. This step trains us to accept everything as holy.

Finally in the tenth step, Prasada, our mind becomes one with god's mind and we experience true joy.

The ability to feel is the most basic and fundamental state of mind we can experience, and it has a great power over us, other people, and nature.

The ability to feel can be developed anytime you have the intention. It's never too late, even if you're old, because this ability is already buried inside of us.

The beginning of meditation: Pratyahara

It's important to master the mind and body training you've learned so far so that you can practice it anytime. Pratyahara enables you to "learn it with your body."

In the beginning, you'll practice doing everything "consciously."

You'll then maintain this awareness until you can do it subconsciously. At that point, you will experience self-control for the first time.

It may help you understand if I use the example of riding a bicycle. When you begin learning to ride a bicycle, you have to be conscious of riding it in order to stay up – but once you get used to it, it doesn't feel like anything. Once you're able to ride it subconsciously, you can ride in the most logical and effective manner.

It's the same with the practice of quieting your breath. In the beginning you have to constantly think "quiet breath" in order to do it, but as you keep doing it, it becomes part of you.

If you change yourself intentionally, even if you want to change, you're basing your actions on ideas you borrowed from someone else. It's as if you've been given orders and become their slave. But if a thought comes to you subconsciously, it's yours at last and no one else's.

Become your own hero

Think of being given orders as the most shameful thing there is. You can't perform well when someone tells you what to do.

In this practice, you become your own hero. You control yourself. If someone gives you orders all the time, you can't think for yourself. So only give yourself orders, discipline and manage yourself.

In order to do this, you have live consciously. I always say to myself, "You, Masahiro Oki, do you think what you're doing is good?" "Just a moment. After some consideration, I think I should do it the other way." Instruct yourself consciously. This is the first step to focusing your mind. It's also called, in philosophical terms, "self-annihilation" or "spiritual state of nothingness." Direct your senses to the way you want to feel, and train until you can experience silence within noise, or feel warmth within cold.

Or try imagining that you don't have parents, even if you do. Imagine you don't have children, even if you do. Imagine you don't have a wife or girlfriend, even if you do. Imagine you don't have money, even if you do, and that you don't have life, even though you do.

By doing this, you naturally create the attitude to deal with whatever happens in the best possible state. You become more aware, more naturally willing to be caring, and more inclined to want to do your best. Practice this kind of attitude every day.

Thinking that you have money makes you restless with worry, insecurity, and doubt. Intentionally separate your awareness from your obsession, and observe your mind and body objectively. Even though you have something, you have nothing. Even though you have nothing, you have something. Place yourself in the extreme opposite state and continue practicing consciously.

Give yourself praise

I enjoy cigarettes and alcohol as much as anyone. But I can always quit. Having control over oneself is a state in which it's okay to drink or not drink.

When I tell people this, they ask me if it works. Some people ask me what they should do to quit smoking. They can't quit because they don't. If they let other people control them, they'll never be able to quit their own cigarettes habit.

People give themselves commands, too. "Let's have only ten cigarettes today." And once you've had the tenth one, it becomes a battle. You can't break the promise you made to yourself.

And here is where you have to draw a clear line: unless you can do that, you are more likely to become your own slave and accumulate more bad habits more. In the yogic dojo, there is no reward or punishment. When someone makes a mistake, I tell them to come to me after they've thought about how they would punish themselves.

Nobody has a right to punish others. Humans are weak animals, so if we have any rights or qualifications at all, it's to help each other. Laws are there to protect the social order, but they're evils that shouldn't have to exist.

You need to praise yourself, too. Falling in love with yourself is the best feeling. It's being given a reward from god. But I know that I don't have the qualification to receive this reward yet. When I do receive it, I will experience the true joy and satisfaction of living this life.

Observe yourself with Pratyahara (Emotion Controlling Autonomic Sadhana Ascetic Training): the Yogic practice of turning the mind to introspection by voluntarily shutting out distractions provided by the senses

I'll now explain the practical methods of Pratyahara (Emotion Controlling Autonomic Sadhana Ascetic Training).

Pratyahara is a form of mind training that teaches you to direct your senses, which normally tend to react to outside stimulation, into your mind, shutting down impressions from the outside world. By consciously unifying your mind in this way, your emotions, thoughts, and actions become more stabilized.

In our lives, we often have a really good day because the weather is great and it feels great. We're very much controlled by simple sensations such as comfort and discomfort.

So we'll begin by focusing our mind inward. However, because it's difficult for a beginner to practice *Pratyahara* on their mind, we begin practicing with physical methods. Here are some of the most common methods practiced in yoga.

Yoni Mudra

Yoni mudra calms your mind and enhances your awareness and concentration. If you practice this for a long time, you'll achieve no-mind.

1. Sit in *Kekka-Fuza* (Padmasana, or Lotus Position) and take a deep breath.
2. In order to shut down your audiovisual functions from the outside world, hold your eyes, ears, and nose. Hold your ears with your thumbs, eyes with your index fingers, nose with your middle fingers, and upper lip with your pinkies.
3. Hold your breath and focus your power in your tanden.
4. Concentrate your awareness on the sound you hear in your ears. You'll realize that the sound changes into different sounds.
5. As you practice this, chant "om" – a yogic sacred sound – as you slowly exhale.
6. Focus your awareness in your tanden.
7. When you can't hold your breath any longer, release your hands and breathe out quietly. Repeat these steps until your mind becomes quiet.
8. Now practice hearing the same sound without holding your ears. If you succeed in paying attention to this sound created with your imagination, hold your ears again and separate your mind from the sound in your ears, shifting your attention to the sound you create with your imagination.
9. If you're successful up to this point, you are able to freely control the function of your mind that goes outward and change its direction inward.

Pratyahara also trains you to pay attention and focus. Therefore, by continuing to practice it patiently, anyone can achieve a state of no-mind. If you can control the function of your mind like this, you won't get disturbed easily.

Now let's start the next meditation practice.

2. BE CREATIVE WITH MEDITATION PRACTICE

Fifth step: Dharana (Unifying Sadhana Ascetic Training)

Humans, when they can collect their power, can live creatively being themselves. The practice to accomplish this can be done by collecting the mind and directing it toward a subject. This is the fifth step, Dharana.

First, you intentionally unify the conscious and subconscious in your mind and bring your entire body together to support it. Then you connect the whole power of your body and mind and train yourself to engage your power at will. The ability to unify the power of body and mind is called psychokinesis. When you think and act upon your psychokinesis, you're totally engaged in the action or committed to it. It's the way to express your power most logically and effectively.

Dharana, which means continuance, is about *Darani* in the Shingon Sect of Japanese Buddhism. One needs to continue some kind of action in order to focus the mind and gather life force energy. In this sect, they practice methods such as continuously watching a mandala or reciting a mantra.

An easy way to do this is to focus all your power into whatever you're doing right now. When you walk, focus on walking. When you read, just become the act of reading itself. Don't think about anything else, because if you do, you and your action split.

When we're worried, humans sometimes get consumed by a thought and can't think of other things. But this isn't focus of mind; rather, it's an attachment. Understand, too, that you can't really concentrate your mind just because you're told to.

In the beginning, doing what you like to do, such as music or sports, can be Dharana. Motorbike riders aren't thinking about other things when they ride their motorbikes. Dancing like crazy at a dance club can be an elementary Dharana. But, just as you practiced in Pratyahara, you have to do this intentionally. Doing what you like subconsciously is simply a bad habit. If you want to quit, you have to be able to quit at your will.

Consciously create a state in which you can be most inspired. Being surprised, touched, pushed, or having a clear purpose would make anyone concentrate and focus. This is a key to studying or working too. When something's unusual, you don't forget it, and you can remember things better when you're in a pinch.

Rather than playing catch mindlessly, intentionally throwing a ball in a different and creative way enables you to concentrate on your throw. Keep asking yourself questions when you're studying. Shine a different light by asking a question such as "What if I think this way?" or "Is there any other way to analyze this?" If you stare at something from a fixed direction, you can't concentrate your mind. Dharana is training yourself to feel, think, and act from as many different angles as you can.

When the conscious and subconscious layers of the mind are unified and the body is cooperative, you achieve a state in which, if you concentrate all your mind, nothing can't be accomplished.

Sixth step: Dhyana (Zen Sadhana Ascetic Training)

When a beginner practices concentration alone, they're constantly tense, creating an imbalance in the mind and body. When body and mind are unified, they're healthy and in good condition, but humans also need relaxation, rest, and sleep. That's where Dhyana and Bhakti, which you're about to practice, come in. *Dhyana* (from Sanskrit "*Dhyāna*," or "*Jhāna*" in *Pāli*, a stage of meditation that is a subset of, and synonymous to, Samādhi) relaxes the body, and detachment relaxes the mind.

In terms of Yin-Yang, unification is Yang and Dhyana and detachment are Yin. In Yang practice you increase tension and gather power, and in Yin practice you release it and relax. The body and mind are most stable when there's a balance between Yin and Yang. And in addition, in order to get to the eighth step, Samadhi, where you and others become one, you have to be able to empty yourself.

Dhyana, which I recite here at the sixth step, is what must have been pronounced "Dzenna" in old Chinese (which later became "Zen" in Japanese), the teaching that later became the basis of Chinese and Japanese Zen Buddhism. It means "ultimate relaxation and stability." In other words, the mind, body, and life are unified and most stable. Your body and mind become clear and you feel refreshed, relaxed, and quiet. This isn't, however, a lack of energy, but rather a state that's very energetic yet relaxed.

We're able to attain the best balance when we do the right action at the right time for the right amount. This is called the Laws of Ki, Do, and Ma (opportunity, degree, and suitable placement). For example, if I make my body sit in the position that's necessary at the moment, my posture is most stable. But in order to do this, you have to discover what you really are. You can't ask other people to tell you what to eat or what kind of job you should get.

Doing Zazen can be Zen Sadhana but you can't just sit in silence. The entire you – your mind, body, and life – have to be sitting. This is difficult without training. For example, imagine that you're sitting down with your legs crossed and you tell yourself, "Don't think of anything. Stay with no thoughts." Would the "self" within you listen to what you say? Your idle thoughts come up even more as you try to get rid of them. It's just like the psychology of wanting to open a door when we're told not to.

When this happens, let the idle thoughts keep coming. Just observe them one by one as they come up. You can apply this idea to help you concentrate your mind. If you don't treat the thoughts as idle thoughts, they're not idle thoughts anymore. It may take a while in the beginning, but in time the amount of idle thoughts that come up will be shorter. Then you'll experience *Zenjo* (*Dhyana/Jhana*) like a blue sky after clouds drift away with the wind. This can be achieved by anyone who tries.

Seventh step: Bhakti
(Faith Sadhana Ascetic Training)

The seventh step, *Bhakti,* is also called *Detachment Sadhana.* In this practice, you train in detachment of mind; in other words, you empty yourself. It's training your mind to be unconditionally "devout."

Subliminally let go of the self that's self-centered and egoistic, and have a mind that doesn't get caught up, fixate, or get led astray. Bhakti is giving yourself to others.

But devotion doesn't mean clinging to something. One principle of yoga is that you alone can save yourself. If a religion is about worshipping in order to make money or pass an exam, it must be an evil creed. It's about business.

Rather, you devote yourself to god, without thinking of loss and profit, and are grateful for everything. In other words, you enter a state of "surrender." Needless to say, you must be diligent to focus yourself to the limit. If you only practice detachment, you're nothing but lazy. To devote yourself is to set an intention to let go of your self-centered selfish mind and give yourself to the truth.

So how do people in the yogic dojo practice devotion to god? Let me explain a bit. First, they submit themselves to their teacher or guru in Hindu. In my dojo, my order is an absolute. My students have to go if I tell them to go, or sit if I tell them to sit. When I say this, they usually complain in the beginning. But I do understand that I'm telling them unreasonable things. I say these things knowing that. Detachment Sadhana is completely without reason.

It's not a practice of obedience, though. It's a practice of devotion. It is rather difficult to empty yourself, but if you don't practice it, you can't attain *Mushi* (selflessness), *Muga* (non-selfhood), or *Munen-Muso* (a serene state of mind without earthly thoughts), or practice *Samadhi,* in which you treat another's mind as your own—because it's only when you're empty that another's mind can come into you. By the same notion, you can't pour water into a cup unless it's empty.

In yoga, you overcome your own difficulties

At my dojo, people often come to me because they've hit the wall in their work and so forth, but I always tell them, "Stop being a wimp." A pianist, for example, comes to the dojo expecting that practicing yoga will help them play the piano better. Yes, they'll be able to play a little better, because they'll be able to relax their shoulders and arms and move their fingers more easily. But even if they get better at yoga, which they began out of dependency, there will be no true music.

Humans always reach their own limit when they commit themselves seriously to something. If they do something as a hobby, they can always change paths, but if it's their life work, things are different. You have to face these walls many times.

You may think a "wall" is a bad thing, but it's not. Hitting the wall is the only opportunity for you to jump onto the next step. If you're not seriously committed, you wouldn't hit the wall. In fact, you should be concerned when you don't hit the wall.

Spontaneously searching for your own limitation is important because that's the beginning of everything. If you hit the wall, you're forced again and again to try to focus your mind. Then when you have no other way and you've done your best, you empty your mind and begin to see the other side of the wall. That's why it's important to discover something you can commit yourself to. If you don't try your best, you can't believe. If you don't think and think, you can't get out of your circle of thoughts.

When people come to my dojo with certain desires, I turn them down. I say, "You can't cure your disease or depression here. Go somewhere else." When the basis is dependency, even if a disease is cured, it's not cured fundamentally. If you want to heal, heal with your own power. When you awaken to it, your way of living will be liberated. Unifying Sadhana is to try to do as much as one can as a human being, and Zen Sadhana and detachment Sadhana is to "surrender to fate."

Next, I'll explain how to practice these three methods in more detail.

How to practice Dharana (Unifying Sadhana Ascetic Training)

You need to do a warm-up before you practice Dharana. There's no specific way to do this, so if you like baseball, you can play catch, or if you practice martial arts, you can perform the kata. You can also sing or laugh. The purpose is to relax the body, though, so don't overdo it.

Dharana (Unifying Sadhana Ascetic Training)

Once you're relaxed, inhale, bring energy to your tanden, and hold the breath. Relax your body as you exhale. As you do so, imagine you are taking the prana, or ki, of the universe into your body, and exhaling it out.

1. Choose a sitting posture that's most comfortable for you from the postures I introduced previously. Stable Sitting Pose (*Siddhasana* for men and *Siddha Yoni Asana* for women) is the most common. In this pose, stand up and turn and twist the body to both sides to find out which side is easier. The pelvis is loose on that side.

2. Bring the heel of that looser side to your perineum, and bring your other foot over the outside of the other leg, keeping it close to the perineum as well.

3. Close your eyes and keep your lower back straight as if you're pushing down on your pelvis. Tighten your stomach and lift your chest. Keep your shoulders parallel, as if you were carrying an egg under your armpits. Tuck in your chin and relax your neck, shoulders, and chest, as if your head were being held up by a string.

4. Push your tongue against the roof of your mouth, tighten your

rectum as you tighten the stomach, lift your upper body, and have use force on the inside of your knees to push against the floor. This will fill your tanden naturally with power. This may feel like too much work at first, but if you do it every day for a week, you will become accustomed to it.

5. Use the power of suggestion to let go of force intentionally. Visualize and tell yourself that your head is relaxed, your hands are relaxed, and so forth, one after another.

6. In the beginning, use the total breathing technique. After a while, total breathing will become more automatic and rhythmic, all the muscles in your body will become unified from the breath, and your breath will become a deep, quiet, and peaceful *Taisoku* Breathing, or Whole Body Breathing (This is a breathing method that mimics the way an embryo breathes in its mother's womb; you gradually make your breathing small and long, eventually decreasing the number of breaths you take to one or two a minute or so. Eventually you breathe as if you were breathing through your navel as an embryo does. This breathing method, also called "pore breathing," can enhance the oxygen exchange capacity of the cells.)

Now, to focus you mind, use the following methods.

Ways to Concentrate Your Mind

Dharana (Unifying Sadhana Ascetic Training) is a method that develops the ability to feel. Animals sustain life though their ability to feel and to react to those feelings. Even when stimulation is present, if there's something wrong with your body, your ability to feel is also off. If that ability is weak, you can get sick easily.

To develop your ability to feel, focus your consciousness on one subject, such as a sound, your breath, an object, or your tanden.

Beginners should choose something simple, such as the ticking of a clock, the smoke from a stick of incense, or a black dot drawn on a wall. As you continue to focus, these things change slightly. The sound of the clock may grow louder or quieter. By paying attention to and being interested in these changes, you will stay focused.

Other methods can include the following.

A. *Bhrukuti* (concentration at the space between the eyes, as if looking up between the eyebrows): In this method, you concentrate on the spot between your eyes. Try to see right between your eyebrows.

B. *Nasa-agra Drishti* (concentration at the tip of the nose, common in Zen schools): In this method, you concentrate on the tip of your nose. This is used in Zen.

C. Shat-ataru (concentration by shifting focus. In this method, often used in Theravada Buddhism, we keep changing the point of concentration from one place to another.): In Hinayana (lesser or small vehicle) Buddhism, the six glands in our body are called chakras. In this method, you change the location of your focus from one charka to the next, from the coccyx through the spine to the crown of the head.

Mantra (holy words / holy sounds)

Vocalize or silently chant the sound aum (sometimes written om), concentrating your mind on the sound. This practice is used in Islam as a way to focus, as well as in China, where it is called *Onmyodo* (rhythmic breathing).

① With your mouth open, make the sound "a." As you do so, arch you back, keeping strength in your lower back and relaxing your hands and body. This helps disperse your body temperature and alkalizes the blood. (When it's hot, we say "ah" or "ah, it's hot," which subconsciously lowers body temperature.)

② Purse your lips and make the sound "o" as you lean forward and tighten your body, keeping you back straight and keeping strength in your arms. This minimizes the diffusion of body heat and makes the blood acidic. (When it's cold, we say "oh, it's cold" or "oh it's freezing".)

③ Make the sound "m" with your lips together. Lower your shoulders, keeping them parallel, and gather energy in your lower abdomen. This naturally fills your tanden with energy and neutralizes the blood. The sound unifies the mind and body and awakens the inner ability.

Repeating the sound aum helps your body maintain balance. As you do so, release your voice from your backbone, shaking your spine from the bottom so that the sound echoes throughout your whole body.

How to practice Zenjo (Dhyana/Jhana) and Detachment Sadhana Ascetic Training

Always practice *Zenjo* and *Detachment Sadhana* after you practice *Dharana* (*Unifying Sadhana*). First, shake or rub your body lightly to loosen it. (This same principle is used when people fall asleep on the train or in a car, or to help children relax by rubbing their head.)

Next, to loosen your mind, tense your body tightly and then relax it all at once. This changing rhythm of tension and relaxation relaxes the mind, in the same way that a timid person becomes bold after experiencing an extreme fear.

As you exhale more deeply, longer, and stronger, both your mind and body begin to loosen and relax. It's the same in daily life, when your breath naturally becomes longer during an after-work smoke, or when, after being in a room with dirty air, you go outside and feel the clean air and find yourself naturally taking a deep breath. A sigh is another kind of relaxing breath.

Here are the methods to use.

Zenjo (Dhyana/Jhana) and Detachment Sadhana Ascetic Training

In the *Stable Sitting Pose* (*Siddhasana* for men and *Siddha Yoni Asana* for women) that you use in *Dharana,* close your eyes and practice the following.

① Tuck in your chin and straighten your spine, turning your eyes inward as if your hair is being pulled upward from your head. This helps your consciousness become clear and your senses sharp. (Conversely, when you jut out your chin and bend your spine, your eyes move forward.)

② Expand your chest sideways to relax your upper body.

③ Push your hips forward, lengthen your abdominal muscles, press your buttocks toward the floor, and lift your upper body. This stabilizes your lower body and gives it more power.

④ Release tension by telling yourself, "Now my head is relaxed," "My hands are relaxed," and so on.

⑤ Your breath should be aligned in a natural rhythm, deep, quiet, and soft. When you reach a point where you don't even feel your own breath, your body will be totally relaxed and your mind empty.

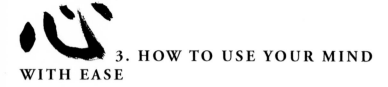

3. HOW TO USE YOUR MIND WITH EASE

Eighth step: Samadhi (Sadhana Ascetic Training)

This practice helps you become one with others.

When you excel at riding a horse, you become one with the horse. You ride in a way that brings out the best of the horse, more so even than when no one is riding it. When this happens, the horse moves in a way that allows the rider to be more stable.

In Samadhi, the human becomes the mind of the horse, and the horse becomes the mind of the human. It is love.

Try practicing Samadhi in your daily life, in your relationships between man and man, man and animal, man and anything. When you release an arrow, make the mind of the bow and arrow yours. You don't play the violin; the violin is played by you. We shouldn't enslave the violin. It's the same with anything, whether a sewing machine or a computer.

One day, a famous Japanese sculptor came to me and said he'd like to give me a sculpture he had recently made. But I refused, saying that I appreciated his generosity but didn't want it. He thought I was just being reserved because it was such a valuable sculpture, but that wasn't the case. I refused because I thought it wasn't really a sculpture. When I told him so, he asked me why.

I answered his question like this: "If you think this is a sculpture, take a look at the pillar over there. On it, there are numerous scratches that children have made with nails. That is carved wood also, but would you call it a sculpture? Of course not. People who have no idea may think this creation of yours is a sculpture, but to me it is just carved wood.

"Real sculpture is carved in the way that makes the material the happiest, by understanding its mind and its desires. Did this wood tell you to carve like this? I suspect that you made up something in your head to make it. Isn't that egoism? You can't ignore the wood.

"A sculpture is already carved in the material. If you can read what the rock wants, or read the wood's mind, you will come to see the form to carve out. Humans are only allowed to carve out the form that is there. Make the mind of the wood yours."

If you do your work in the way that makes it happy, your work will treat you kindly. If you do your work in the way that makes it unhappy, your work will tell you so by making you tired.

If you work to make your work happy, you will enjoy your work. It will give you joy. You create the joy, but others give you the joy. It is will of others to thank you, and you cannot force it. It is your duty to create a situation or condition that causes them to thank you.

Samadhi means to become one with others

In Samadhi, somebody else's mind becomes your mind as it is. Your mind becomes somebody else's mind as it is. Their desires become your desires. Therefore, when asked a question, although my fundamental and underlying idea of the answer remains the same, I try to answer in superficially different ways according to the personality of the person asking or the situation at the time. It is because I would like to tell the person what they need to hear at the moment in the way that suits them.

When parents talk to their children, they need to speak in a way that makes children want to listen—to understand the mind of their children and speak in their tongue. You need to explain things so that children can understand and be satisfied and happy. It's important that your children feel grateful when you tell them your story.

Parents need to ask themselves whether they scold or praise their children out of self-complacency. If they speak for the sake of their own convenience, their children will either rebel or become dependent.

How do you become a child's mind? By remembering your own childhood. Try to dig through your memories to find out what helped you among all praising or scolding.

Just a little praise can make people confident in what they do. That's even truer for children. But if you compliment your children just because it's easier for you to do so, it can make them overconfident or proud. And when you scold children for your own satisfaction or for no reason at all, it will only cause them to rebel or act perversely. However, if you become the child's mind and scold them in the way they understand, they grow with your words as a guide.

To think as if your mind is others'

Making what you are committed to doing a "do-the way of'" leads to Samadhi. Turn cooking into "cooking-do", baseball into "basball-do", tennis into "tennis-do". Even walking can be "walking-do". "Do" may seem difficult to achieve, but it isn't. There's not even a teacher.

Turning everything into a "do" is my philosophy. It's the key to living your life the way it fits you.

Have you questioned the word Ikebana, which is usually translated "flower arrangement" in English but literally means "giving life to flowers?"

How does cutting flowers in nature to display in a room, shortening their life span, become an act of "giving life to flowers?"

When you look at the art of giving life to flowers as kado, or "the way of flowers," flowers are not considered just decoration; rather, they are literally given life. Flowers live for a week if they are rooted in the dirt, but usually die in three days if they're cut. But if they are arranged with the mind of kado, they can stay alive for ten days to two weeks.

In order to do this, make the mind of the flowers your own. Support the mind of the flower, which wants to live. The principle of living is the principle of balance, of harmonizing the things that are antagonistic to unify and balance them. This is the work of universe, earth, and man. Kado is about learning the mind of the universe and the earth through giving life to flowers in order to master the principle of life and acquire the mind of love.

Ninth step: Buddhi (Buddha Nature Enlightenment Sadhana Ascetic Training)

Buddha nature is what the religion that was born in India set as the foundation of its view of the world and humanity. It is a practice that develops a mind that sees and respects the divinity within ourselves and others. By this practice alone, we can make humanity holy.

In yoga, too, it is our principle of life to see and treat ourselves and others as divine. We do this by joining our palms together and worshipping. In this practice, also called *Sacred Heart Sadhana: Cultivation of the Sacred and Holy Nature in You*, you learn to see everything as precious, good, and valuable and train to make your mind holy.

Let's take business, for example. Suppose I open a store and have many products. That alone doesn't make me a merchant. The products are not there for me to use. It's the customers who use the products. The products are not mine, but theirs. In other words, the customers are the heroes. If a customer comes, it means a hero comes, because god sent them in order to make me a merchant. Therefore, it is as if god came to you.

The products, too, are precious. They make me a merchant and create a connection between me and the customer, or god. They are not just things, but benefactors. These benefactors make me who I am, make the customer who they are, and create a connection to god. Therefore, the products are gods too.

Neither is the store mine. It's a store for the customers, and I'm just a guard protecting their products. I simply try my best to choose and keep products that make them happy.

This attitude of service is important. It's not limited to merchants. When you acquire a viewpoint of gratitude and humbleness, your way of seeing and feeling becomes different from the worldly mind that's caught up with loss and profits.

Many people with physical or mental illnesses come to me every day. They are sent to me by god. "I'll leave these people with you to help solve their problems. This is for you as well. If these people aren't saved, you won't be saved."

Because I think this way, I'm accepting of everyone. I try my best. It's not about profit or reward. It is my god-given duty, and these are the people that god sent me.

You can live easily with a mind like this

The motto of my dojo is "gratitude, penitence, lower seat/sitting low, service, and a mind of love."

Penitence means feeling guilty and, as I understand it, feeling responsible, not just regretful. It's feeling gratitude and acting on that feeling.

Our food, for example, was once alive. When I eat it, I kill it, and its life sustains my life. When we eat pork, we killed a pig, even though we didn't directly kill it ourselves.

We kill honorable daikon radish, carrots, sardines, and other foods to sustain our lives as we consume theirs. If you accept this with honesty, feelings of gratefulness, acknowledgement, and apology naturally spring from your heart. These feelings awaken you to a mind that wants to repay the favor. If you feel this way, there's no other way for you to live but to live your life lively and to its full extent.

This is penitence, and without it you won't have gratitude or the willingness to serve.

Lower seat/sitting low is a state of mind that doesn't do someone a favor out of condescension, but instead feels grateful. If you do something out of condescension—thinking "I did this for you," like the mafia—even if you don't say it out loud, it's called upper seat/sitting high.

I've never become angry even if someone I took care of turned their back on me. It was my privilege to look after them. I gained joy in doing so.

What's important is having a mind that's satisfied just by being able to love someone. That is the mind of lower seat/sitting low. If you love someone because you want something in return, it's a mind of upper seat/sitting high, and it inevitably causes hate, anger, grudges, complaint, and dissatisfaction, which keeps you frustrated. Why don't we stop such pointless mind games? When you become aware of this, a mind of lower seat/sitting low begins.

I didn't have a mind of lower seat/sitting low in the beginning. I acquired it gradually as I disciplined myself. I had more a mind of upper seat/sitting high in the beginning. In fact, probably because I experienced the extreme of the mind of upper seat/sitting high, I came to appreciate the value of mind of lower seat/sitting low. There may not be anyone who has mind of lower seat/sitting low first. It's difficult for any of us to commit to work unless we have desires. Down the road, when you experience the extreme, you begin to see what mind of lower seat/sitting low is about. So I won't tell you to have mind of lower seat/sitting low now. I just want you to know that there is such a state of mind and you can truly live easily once you acquire it.

Tenth step: Prasada

Prasada is a Hindi word meaning true joy, and practicing Prasada is training to experience everlasting joy, also called Ananda, or Ascetic Training through Delight Sadhana.

When you experience the state of Samadhi and Buddhi, Prasada will flow out of your mind and body endlessly. It is truly a paradise on earth, a state of the enlightenment of Buddha where everything is good, joy, and light. Buddha was enlightened through Prasada practice.

What is true joy? My understanding is that it is a state where my joy, your joy, and god's joy come together. If only I am happy, or you are happy, or only you and I are happy, it's not Prasada. We cannot call it Prasada unless god is happy too.

Prasada is the joy of holy men, and it exists only in holy lands. My mind won't be able to feel the joy of god unless it becomes god's mind. If you can make god's will your will, you are one with god. Etsu, an act of feeling delighted, in truth means eternal joy.

People can taste Prasada when they acquire the compassion of god, which is beyond human compassion. At that moment, people experience the blessings of the entire universe and its joy.

I consider this tenth step the only yoga.

Man is part of nature

We should live with thoughts that satisfy everyone, that everyone agrees with and is happy about. That's the will of god. That's what man wishes for and nature aspires to as well. I think that living this way is a universal wish that resides in every life force.

God is something that our entire society agrees upon, despite individual differences. There can be objection, of course. I'm not saying that everyone has to agree, and that those who disagree are heretics. Every man is different; therefore it's unnatural to think that everyone has to be exactly the same.

A force that connects man and man, man and the universe, in a place of oneness, despite these little differences—that's what I call "god." God that exists in all things is also within us. You can see god. When you discover god within yourself, you can see god in others, and see the mind of god in others' minds. The connection between the god and the self is religion.

All things are seen the way you see them, and become what you treat them to be. This is the principle of "what goes around comes around," or *Sangai-Isshin*. Sangai is *Tridhātu* in Sanskrit, and means the three realms of desire (*kāmadhātu*), form (*rūpadhātu*), and formlessness (*ārūpyadhātu*). The meditations of form within the realm of form are related to the Buddhist view of the three poisons of the mind: greed (lust, desire, etc.), aversion (hatred, anger, etc.), and ignorance (delusion, illusion, etc.). *Isshin* means One Heart/Mind. Therefore, *Sangai-Isshin* means that all three realms are phenomena that are reflected in our mind/heart and hence, outside of our mind/heart, do not exist. This could also be called "the world is created by the mind." One of the great things about yoga is that it teaches that god exists within ourselves, and we need to look for it. The training of mind and body to see god is the only yogic practice. When every single man is awakened to oneness, the entire universe will sympathize with us and praise us.

What I call "god" is also the will of the universe – a life force or force of creation in nature. The destructive force in nature is just one aspect of the creative force. You can see this in the transition of the seasons. Spring, the season of regeneration and rebirth, comes only after harsh winter, the season of destruction and death. Therefore winter is not really a season of death; it is hiding the seeds of life. The seeds of life exist inside the bark of the trees or underneath the ground. They hibernate during the winter, awaken in the spring, bloom in the summer, and ripen in the fall. This pattern is deeply connected to the cycle of all matter, the revolution of the stars and the universe.

I feel the will of the universe in this. When we see the cycle of the four seasons, it seems to portray how human life should be. The ideal way to live is to know the will of the universal life force, or god, and to live according to it. That's how a person makes their life their own.

The law of nature and the law of the universe are the mind of god. And the mind of god is love. And god's will allows everything to coexist and flourish together. Only through the harmony of every existence in the world can we realize each other's joy of life.

The spirit of yoga is connection with each other, and the practice of yoga is actually living up to this in one's life. Therefore, we can conclude that yoga is a practice that reflects the religious mind in daily life.

You will naturally know the will of god if you observe the way of nature – because we humans are part of nature as well.

Epilogue

CREATE YOUR FUTURE WITH YOGA

How I found yoga

I was eight years old and in second grade when I first learned about yoga. At that time, Bishop Ottama, who was known as the father of independence in the country formerly called Burma, visited my house. My parents had told me stories of Buddha, Jesus Christ, and Muhammad. My household was filled with a religious atmosphere.

The bishop stayed at my house for four or five days, and I had the opportunity to ask him many questions.

"How did Buddha become such a great master?" I asked.

The bishop kindly answered, "Because he practiced yoga."

That was the first time I had heard the word yoga, so I asked him what it was. The bishop's answer was something like this:

There are two kinds of "teaching": *Kengyo* (the opposite/antonym of *mikkyo* or Vajrayana Buddhism and Tantric Buddhism), which honors people, and esoteric teaching, which leads people to enlightenment. *Kengyo* has texts that preach its teachings, and the monks and priests can teach you intelligibly. However, there are no teachers or textbooks in esoteric teachings. Yoga is esoteric.

I was surprised to hear this. How does one study without a teacher or textbook?

"Think," he said. "What would you do if you had to learn in such a situation?"

If there is nothing else to rely on, you can only touch it with your hands, see it with your own eyes, walk on your own feet, think with your own head. When I answered this way, he said "Yes. That's what esoteric teaching is."

You become your own student and teacher. You make everything your teacher. You treat everyone as a benefactor. Take wherever you are as your school. Take every connection that's given to you as a textbook. The way of self-realization—to find out how much you can learn and how much you can act on in your lifetime—is yoga. So it is hard to describe.

The reason we don't teach it in a simple or easy way is because if we do, people pretend to understand and don't work hard, or don't think for themselves.

When someone is dependent, they become self-protective and

don't do anything on their own, even if they have talent. When you're dependent, your desire can build up, leading you in the wrong direction, where you're more nervous, excited, caught up, and stuck.

The basics of yoga

When I said, "I understand now. It means I have to work hard," the bishop shook his head and said: "It's not just about working hard. Do you think it's all the same whether you walk with your eyes closed or open? When your eyes are closed and you have no idea where you're going, you get lost. It's important to walk with your eyes open.

"Everything has the potential to be positive or negative. If you work hard positively, the result will be positive, but if you work hard negatively, the result, in contrast, will be miserable.

"I'll teach you the most important thing you need to master yoga. It's not something I should teach, but for a little child like you, I will. You've learned so much from your teachers, parents, and books. You should know a little about what's good and what's bad."

"Yes, I do. I know a little," I said.

"Practice it," said the bishop. "What you find to be good, or are taught is good, act upon. Make these things yours and master them. In Japanese, you call this shitsuke (discipline), don't you? That's yoga."

In this way, Bishop Ottama taught me the basics of yoga, which for a child like me was easy to understand.

Life yoga that I learned from Master Gandhi

In 1939, when World War II was about to break out, I was chosen to be a special secret agent of the General Staff Office and sent first to Mongolia and then to the Middle East.

On my way to Arabia, I stopped in India and went to visit Master Gandhi, with a letter of referral from Bishop Ottama. Just as I had asked Bishop Ottama, I asked him, "How did Buddha and Jesus come to be called yogi of love?" His answer was the same as the bishop's.

Master Gandhi said, "We call Buddha Sakyamuni Buddha because it means he Sokushin-Jobutsu, meaning, in Buddhism, that a person becomes enlightened and becomes Buddha while retaining his or her own corporal body, or reached enlightenment through yogic meditation practice."

Muni means someone who has practiced perfectly, mastered meditation, and developed the true nature of Buddha. Buddha means someone whose true Buddha nature—a quality found only in humans—is completely functional.

True Buddha nature is a condition in which one can understand and deal with all things in a holy state. It is about becoming a true holy person who can respect themselves and others. Someone who has gone from the mundane world to the holy world is called Buddha, or hotoke/butsu.

In short, yogic practice teaches the theory and methods of how to be *hotoke/butsu*. Jesus and Jina (the founder of Jainism) practiced the same methods as Buddha. So you can see that yogic practice is about developing one's true Buddha nature, or a path to enlightenment.

I came to be a peaceful thinker, a liberalist, because I was able to study and practice yoga. Master said he learned yoga when he was in South Africa. When I asked him to teach me its theory and method, he said "I cannot teach yoga because it's an esoteric teaching. I am not a master of yoga itself, so I cannot teach you theories, or even think about it. However, I live my life as yogic practice, so observe how I live and get hints for yourself." And he gave me a room near his.

There I had an opportunity to observe how Master Gandhi lived. The system at Oki Yoga Dojo is based on his way of living.

A day of yoga

What I came to understand as I copied the way Master Gandhi lived is that yoga is about following the law of nature, and that following the law of nature means transforming oneself and continuing to evolve the mind, while at the same time maintaining a balanced and stable way of life.

For example, when we sleep, the functioning of our parasympathetic nervous system is enhanced. Blood is alkalized, food is transformed into nutrition, and physical fatigue is cured. When we're awake, our system balances itself through the opposite functions.

Therefore, we need a method that enhances the functioning of the sympathetic nervous system and our ability to eliminate waste.

Master Gandhi practiced breathing, went jogging (walking or running) to warm the body, and then bathed in cold water to stimulate the body. The purpose of all this is to maintain balance by providing opposite kinds of stimulation: from sleeping to awakening, from parasympathetic nerves to sympathetic nerves, from acetylcholine stimulation to adrenalin stimulation, and from warm stimulation to cold stimulation.

Afterwards, he practiced meditation every day. His meditation practice began with mind concentration, followed by bhakti practice. This was his way of seeking relaxation following tension, and of using his head after using his body, in order to balance and stabilize throughout the day.

I also experienced fasting for the first time at Master Gandhi's, because he told me that we humans tend to eat too much. Fasting helps us maintain balance.

But one day Master Gandhi told me not to copy others. He said, "You can copy the principle, but not the methods. You have your own way of doing things, and you have to find it. If you don't find your way, you can't experience stability.

"How you sit, how you stand, how you run, how you eat. Discovering how to apply yourself to be the best you can be, how to use yourself in a way that makes your life force happy, how to use your body, how to nurture your mind, and how to live—it's all about stabilizing yourself. This is yoga."

The secret of yoga

I also trained with a Tibetan Buddhist monastery, a secret community of Islam called the Darwish group. I can't talk here about what I learned there, but it was a very harsh ascetic training.One aspect of this training was on concentrating the mind. I learned that by intentionally concentrating my attention by repeating a mantra, I could enter a state of no thoughts while remaining in an optimally tense condition, and I was able to enter a state in which I could let go of myself.

I learned about no thoughts, no ego, no mind, where you somehow let go of everything. This can't be achieved by trying, only by repeatedly doing one thing. If you practice concentration at the same time, you can attain the phenomenon of higher vibration as a byproduct. In addition, your ability to receive and sense will be enhanced through the practice of bhakti, and as a result it's possible to obtain telepathic or clairvoyant ability.

During this trip, I was locked up in a prison in Iran. In the same cell was an archbishop of Islam. He told me what faith is truly about, and true meditation practice. Faith is a state in which you totally abandon your desires and conditions, and surrender and receive whatever is given. I learned to take every fate as god's will.

When you're in a state of surrender, you know that everything is god's teaching and god's love. You experience true gratitude for the first time, and achieve real peace of mind. You understood the Prasada, in which you accept everything as joy. *Samadhi* is making another's mind yours, and becoming one with others. As long as you're caught up in yourself, you can't accept the reality of others. But if you let go of your ego, others naturally come into you. You can understand others like yourself.

In the end, what is yoga? Fundamentally, there is no special thought or practice of yoga. Yoga is a word, a Hindu expression of training or education that combines discipline, practice, and mastery. Yoga merely teaches the basic practices of various religions and sects, and preaches the path to oneness of god and human.

Therefore, the self-development and enlightenment that holy people such as Buddha, Jesus Christ, and Muhammad, and Dogen, Shinran, and Kukai (famous and revered founders of their own Buddhist sects in Japan), as well as others practiced is yoga.

I'll continue to search for it and preach it.

MASAHIRO OKI (1921-1985)

Born in 1921, he spent much of his life for training or sadhana path of training. Oki studied Chinese medicine, Taoism and Zen in China in 1938 and then studied Tibet Buddhism by exploring into the deep area in Mongolia and Tibet. He also went to Arabic countries, Iran and India where he trained in various Yoga ashrams with studying Brahmanism.

After he came back to Japan, he graduated from Osaka University of Foreign Studies in 1943, and again went to China, South East Asia and Middle East to study medicine and religion including Taoism, Hinduism, Islamism and Judaism. In 1951 he went to India and Pakistan as a representative to UNESCO Japan, and volunteered and lived in Gandhi's ashram. He learned Gandhi's philosophy is based on Yoga and became an enthusiastic seeker of the truth till his death.

Oki opened a Yoga training ashram which at the time was the only one in Japan and established Japan Yoga Association in 1958. He traveled to Europe and gave lectures in France and other countries, followed by the long lecture series about Zen and Buddhism in the U.S. in 1962. He received diploma in Medicine and Philosophy from India and Switzerland.

He interpreted Yoga into modern thinking and integrated medicine, Zen, and Japanese philosophy and established a unique system called OKIDO Yoga. Through his long training experience and an abundance of knowledge, he improved the ways of meditation, and invented unique a technique of corrective poses to "The balance," "The imbalance of Body, Mind and Spirit." He also educated and trained many disciples from all over the world and healed numerous people. He died in Italy in 1985.

KAZUKO TATSUMURA HILLYER

Kazuko Tatsumura Hillyer was born to a distinguished old family of silk in Kyoto Japan and graduated from Toho conservatory of Music in Tokyo. In 1961 she came to United States as a pianist invited by the Boston Symphony. She studied at Boston University, New York University, and received a PhD in Oriental Medicine from NY State University and the International Academy of Education in Tokyo.

From 1968 to 1992, she promoted cultural exchange from East to West and vice versa; and in 1970s and during the 80s, became a world famous impresario producing 2,000 events each year all over the world. In this connection in 1972, she went to Dahlamsala to find the lost Tibetan Folk Opera, and met His Holiness, the Dalai Lama, with whom she remains a lifelong friend. HH gave her the Tibetan name, *Tenzin Yangchen*. In 1974, she arranged and funded personally the tours of the Folk Opera of Tibet to the West, and contributed the forming of the Tibet Performing Arts Center in Dhalamsala.

She retired from the field of promotions in 1992. She received many medals and honors from different countries.

Her tireless lifelong work in the philanthropic field is vast and well known ranging from Save the Beacon Theater, Save the Boat People, Help the Homeless, Natural Disaster Relief, Aids, and HIV positive children in Africa, etc., but her dedicated work for Tibet and Tibetan children remains very strong in her heart. She writes books and lectures and works with people for holistic health.